Save Our Selves and Protect Planet Earth

Paperback 145 pages
ISBN: 978-9403641720
Draft2Digital ISBN: 979-8201209445
Barnes & Noble, Kobo, Apple, Amazon
E-book
Draft2Digital ISBN: 979-8201328382
Kindle, Kobo, Bol.com

Travel videos on You Tube/Peter Holst MD

Index

Preface

In part one you will see how diseases and global warming are result of exploitation of livestock and nature. Violence has been the inescapable companion of history since time immemorial and is the basis of our existence. It is reflected in how man (but actually all that lives) feeds on what lives and exploits its surroundings. Prevent a repetition of the fall of Easter Island.

For half a century, Mother Earth has given man dominion over his own reproduction and the reproduction of all animals and plants on Earth. We are therefore indebted to repair the damage we cause. Meat and eggs for consumption are now exclusively produced by artificial insemination and with breeding and incubators. African swine fever, annual Influenza viruses and Coronavirus pandemics are the result of diseases in animals that can also pass to humans.

Our distant ancestors are the great apes. We cannot deny this origin. If humanity returns from omnivore to fructivore with food consisting of vegetables, fruits, beans, nuts and the occasional glass of wine, pandemic zoonoses, further increase in cancer cases, and catastrophic global warming will be spared.

Part 2 describes how the Earth can be protected from overconsumption and exhaustion. Abolition of slavery for consumption animals and optimal use of the abundance of energy that the sun gives us are indispensable to this. Development aid should go hand in hand with aid to reduce overpopulation in parts of the world with extreme population growth.

Part three describes how we can protect ourselves from diseases that pass from poultry and other livestock to humans and how we can grow old in a healthy way.

People who consume more animal protein have fewer antibodies, even with a small amount of animal protein. The elderly, in particular, develop diseases that arise from diet that reduces immune response and antibody formation.

Part One – WWIII, our fight against the animals

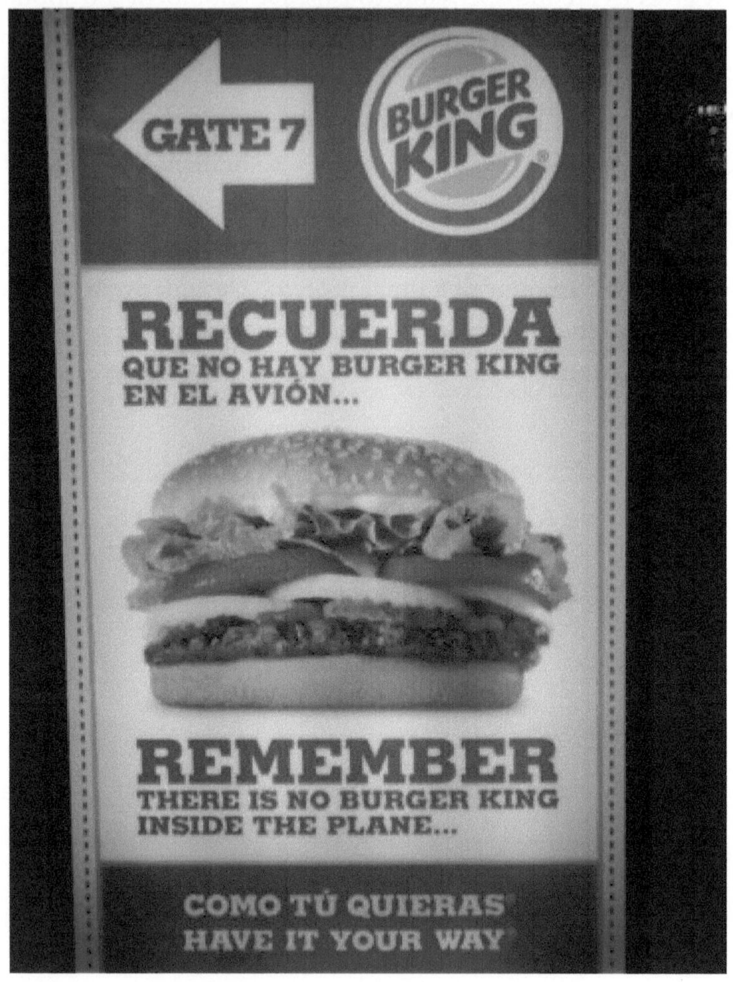

Mass consumption of cheap burgers and flop chickens

Phase 1 of the battle. A bacterial army came from the steppes

The first pandemic was a bacterial pandemic, the bubonic and pneumonic plague in the early Middle Ages (14th century) as a result of the roasting and trading of steppe marmots from Mongolia. The pneumonic plague killed 50% of the European population in the 14th century. The plague bacteria have spread by rats, lice and fleas from the marmot fur.

Phase 2. Viruses and bacteria went to war together

The Spanish flu of 1918-1919 was a virus and bacterial pandemic. The Influenza A (avian) virus caused a flu epidemic in Fort Riley, Kansas, USA. In this fort they bred chickens and pigs for the soldiers. A cook may be infected with the virus. By mutation, the virus was able to cause infection from person to person. Influenza virus (H1N1) was transferred to Europe through millions of deaths via the troop transports of WWI.

The majority of the flu pandemic deaths of 1918-1919 were directly the result of secondary pneumonia caused by common bacteria in the upper respiratory tract.

Data from the subsequent pandemics of 1957 and 1968 are consistent with these findings.

Morens DM, Taubenberger JK, Fauci AS. Predominant Role of Bacterial Pneumonia as a Cause of Death in Pandemic Influenza: Implications for Pandemic Influenza Preparedness. J Infect Dis. 2008; 198 (7): 962–70

Phase 3. Viruses and bats, the flying rats, go to war together

A subsequent pandemic (WHO 1980) was the HIV-1 virus pandemic due to the trade and sale and consumption of chimpanzee bush meat.

Since then, HIV / AIDS has resulted in an estimated 65 million infections and 25 million deaths. Especially in Africa.

This was followed by the Ebola virus pandemic, also due to the consumption of bush meat and dried bats.

Phase 4. The smallest bacteria go to war from bird cages

After the abolition of slavery, the trade in exotic animals and birds, parrots and songbirds has become the new business model. As a result, avian flu and the quartering of bacteria such as Chlamydia pneumoniae in the respiratory tract of humans. Man is used as a host.

Phase 5. Leukemia viruses (ALV and BLV) spread across our food

These viruses use human cells as hosts to multiply. The spread of these viruses is responsible for the recent increase in colon and breast cancer (more about this in the relevant chapter). Since the mid-20th century, more and more megafarms have been growing where pigs, cows and rabbits are bred exclusively through artificial insemination.

Phase 6. Corona viruses compete from wet markets

Influenza viruses and coronaviruses are distributed year after year mainly from chicken farms, pig fattening farms and wet markets in South East Asia where animals are slaughtered and traded alive.

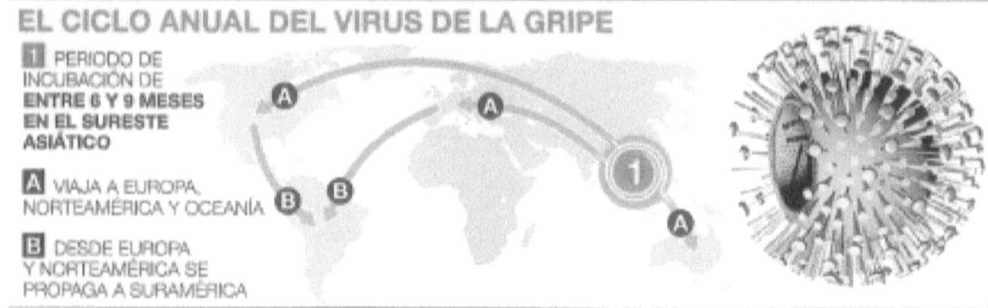

Annual cycle of Flu viruses

In March 2019 the author returned from a cruise in SE Asia, the spice route, and we were in Guangzhou (Canton) for a few days. On arrival at the airport here our temperature was measured and a woman with a fever was discovered and taken for quarantine. Years before the outbreak of COVID-19, since the SARS epidemic, temperature measurement and masks were already practiced in South East Asia in the fight against Coronaviruses!

Coronaviruses spread like nail bombs in humans and cause many deaths from pneumonia. Bats and rodents are carriers of these diseases. Where rats and mice used to transmit diseases, the flying rats (bats) are now the cause of this corona virus pandemic, which comes from wildlife in markets where the animals are traded alive.

It was not until the mid-twentieth century that life on earth got the reproductive processes under control

The first life forms were found in the Pacific region. 400 million years ago Pan Gaia was surrounded by Pan Ocean. The earth was a huge pancake. Life on Earth has evolved Eastward under the influence of gravity, the Earth's rotation and sunrise. Multicellular organisms, fish, marine iguanas and amphibians have emerged from the primordial soup. Dinosaurs, birds, mammals, and monkeys evolved on the land of Pan Gaia. Great apes, homo erectus and homo sapiens originated in Central Africa and Asia.

Homo sapiens has achieved greater manual dexterity in the East African area. Man is the only mammal who can place the thumb opposite the other fingers and make a precision grip with his hands. The more those hands could do, the more successful their owners were, so this evolutionary development created an increasing concentration of nerves and high-precision muscles in the thumb and fingers. The brain grew with it. As a result, people can perform very complex tasks with their hands. Modern man is the first living being who gained control over his own reproduction.

This was followed by control over animal reproduction by applying artificial insemination to the livestock on a large scale

Meat and eggs for consumption in factory farming are exclusively produced by artificial insemination or using incubators.

Coronavirus, African Swine Fever, Bovine Leukemia Virus, Avian Leukemia Virus are the result of diseases in animals that can also pass to humans. More than 300 million farm animals in the EU spend their entire life in a cage. The coronavirus pandemic and the worldwide lock down has shown how fragile society really is.

Meat and dairy consumption continue to rise worldwide, wiping away wildlands, bringing us into contact with potentially dangerous viruses. The world is in lock down and our knowledge and insights are increasing rapidly. The earth has shaped human and we are therefore indebted to our natural environment.

The viruses and bacteria, teach us humans to be careful in our dealings with our fellow mammals. If we do not or insufficiently, we will experience a lot of damage, fear and grief as we already experienced in the Corona year 2020. If we remain stubborn and negligent, we will pay heavily as a species and as individuals. Then it may turn out that we are eventually beaten by the little ones!

Humanity has increasingly come to regard the earth as its exclusive property. Including an increasing portion of the wilderness. We see how the world's population grew and grew, and how almost no one thought about sacrificing their acquired right to a daily piece of meat, resulting in an enormous burden on the environment. All animals have to make do with less and less living space.

Large carnivores - such as the lion - are becoming increasingly rare in the wild, because thanks to humans there is less and less habitat for them and their prey. Tropical forests are being cut down worldwide for soy and palm oil plantations. The soy in turn serves for the food supply of our intensive livestock farming. As a result, on the one hand, the CO2 uptake due to the loss of tropical forest decreases and, on the other hand, the soy through livestock farming causes CO2 to increase. Our planet cannot cope with consumption of meat, there is no room for it. It is high time for people to change their eating habits and to stop trading exotic animals.

Zoonoses

SARS

The SARS epidemic led to about 8,000 infections between November 2002 and July 2003. Nearly eight hundred people died. SARS has spread to more than thirty countries, including countries in Europe. Outside of China, Hong Kong, Canada, Taiwan and Singapore were hit hardest. In China almost all provinces were affected. The Netherlands remained free of SARS. Guangdong Province (Canton) was the focus of this pandemic in 2002. The breeding, trading and eating of civets has been banned there since January 2004. However, recent inspections have shown that civets are still traded there by restaurants, including in Hubei (Wuhan) province.

Coronaviruses and pneumonia

Three new viruses that cause dangerous pneumonia and death in this relatively young century:

- SARS virus that emerged in China in 2002 and was spread via the civet
- MERS virus has come from dromedaries since 2012
- SARS coronavirus II that caused the COVID 19 pandemic

The History of the Corona Outbreak in China

It all started in 2007 with a pandemic of African swine fever (African Swine Fever or ASF) when it entered Georgia (in the Eurasian region of the Caucasus), probably caused by feeding local pigs with ASF virus contaminated offal. including pig remains unloaded from a ship arriving from West Africa. Since then, it has spread across much of Eurasia, eventually infecting pigs and wild boars. The most recent further spread took place in India. The pandemic of African swine fever will be even worse this year (2020) than in 2019, experts say, warning that the spread of the virus, which is highly contagious and deadly for pigs, continues.

With global attention to the human viral pandemic of COVID-19, concerns are growing that countries are being distracted and not focusing enough on stopping the spread of swine fever.

The ASF virus is a much 'stronger' virus than Covid-19 because it can survive for weeks and months in the environment and in processed meats. ASF kills nearly 100% of the animals it infects. The virus has been around for nearly 100 years. in circulation, but no vaccine has yet been developed against it.

ASF virus outbreaks have occurred in multiple provinces of China since August 2018. At the end of 2018, the total number of animals culled was 650,000. China's pig herd, by far the largest in the world, was then estimated at 360 million animals. The number of pigs was almost halved by the end of 2019 due to an epidemic of the ASF virus at the largest pork producer in the world. About 200 million pigs were culled or died as a result of the disease, which reduced pork production by 40%. Production may take more than 5 years to recover to previous levels before the deadly outbreaks due to a lack of solutions to prevent the disease and lack of capital to start new pigs.

Currently, the major reservoirs of the virus are located mainly in China, Vietnam, the Philippines and much of Eastern Europe. The disease has now also spread to Papua New Guinea for the first time.

There are concerns that China is reporting the data for 2020 too rosy. "We see ASF here every week," said Wayne Johnson, veterinarian with the agricultural services company Enable Agricultural Technology Consulting, based in Beijing.

County officials are told not to report. China's policy has now moved from culling to controlling and learning to live with it. The benefit the ASF epidemic has had on the results of pig producers in China adds another interesting dimension to the story. They have already learned to live with the disease in the country and have started to benefit enormously from the higher pork price as a result of the reduced supply. Profits continue to increase at the top Chinese producers such as WH Group, Wens and Muyuan. Pig producers in the US and Europe are growing fears that it is only a matter of time before the disease reaches their swine herds.

At the end of 2019, there was a first outbreak of a new corona virus in Wuhan. The Corona SARS 2 virus has passed from animal to human on a market in the Chinese metropolis of Wuhan. In the live animal market there, exotic animals such as snakes, turtles, bats, foxes and porcupines are sold for consumption. Civets are also still intensively bred, as has been shown by circulating price lists.

The virus is housed and spread by bats, which are cooked alive for soup in China and elsewhere in the world. It is unfortunate that the Year of the Rat 2020 in China is kicking off with a new coronavirus epidemic spread by bats known as the flying rats. After the 2013 SARS epidemic, which spread from Hong Kong, Chinese virologists previously warned that bat-borne coronaviruses would reappear to trigger the next outbreak of the disease. China is a hot spot. Bats are an incredibly diverse group that make up a quarter of all mammals, rodents make up 50 percent, and we humans are among the remaining 25% of mammals. Bats live on every continent, in close proximity to people and farms. The bats' ability to fly provides them with a wide range of habitats, which helps spread viruses. Their stools and urine can spread disease. Bats are the only flying mammals, they devour disease-causing insects by the ton, and they are essential for the pollination of many fruits, such as bananas, avocados and mangoes. Bats are home to a higher proportion of pathogens that pass from animals to humans than any other mammal.

On January 26, 2020, this COVID-19 already caused 2,751 confirmed infections with 56 deaths in China. The virus had already spread to a dozen countries. As of March 4, 2020, there were 80,409 cases, with 3,285 deaths and a spread to 86 countries.

Stopping the sale of wildlife in markets is essential to contain future outbreaks of disease passing from animals to humans.

- **The decision, taken by China's National People's Congress on February 24, 2020, states that the illegal consumption and trade in wild animals will be "severely punished", as will the hunting, trade or transport of wild animals for consumption, is more necessary than ever**

Most Covid-19 infections were in North Brabant, Netherlands

It seems like a big mystery: the corona outbreak in North Brabant. The province is increasingly developing into a source of fire for the virus in the Netherlands. Why most people got infected here?

A year ago, we were at a wedding party near Eindhoven. I walked outside with the idea to enjoy a clear evening. The sky was so polluted with dust that no stars were visible, and there was a pungent smell of neighboring pig fattening farms. How is the indoor air quality in the houses of the many pigeon fanciers, goat breeders, pig farmers and mink farmers? In a bad indoor climate, flu will spread quickly to family members and friends. How is the indoor climate in the many pig slaughterhouses where temperature fluctuates, needs to be worked quickly in a noisy environment and often shout at each other?

During the carnival in North Brabant, the corona virus entered a melting pot of visitors. The risk of contamination is particularly high within banquet halls and bars.

In Germany and the United States also many workers in slaughterhouses and meatpacking industries have proven to be infected with Covid-19 from March to June 2020.

On the accompanying map there is more particulate matter in the air in the red places. In North Brabant this is caused by the many pig stables, the goat breeders, the many bird breeders and the mink farms.

Particulate matter 2.5 and Covid-19 cases

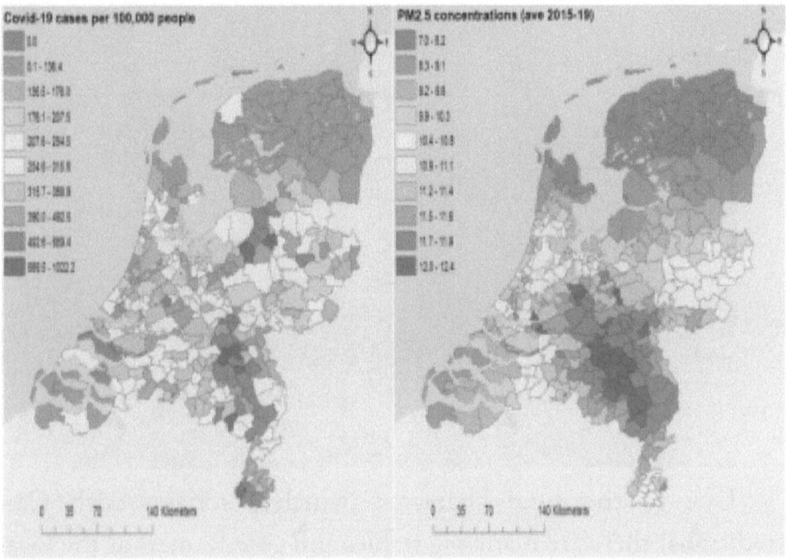

In late February and early March each year carnival celebrations attract thousands of people to street parties and parades – 2020 was no exception, so does that explain the rapid spread of COVID-19 in North Brabant?

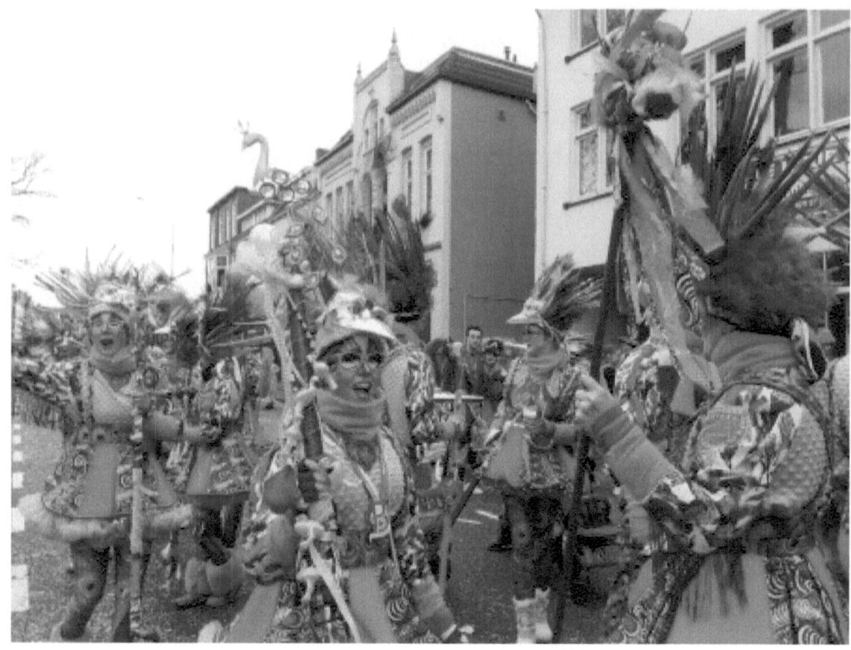

Due to the rural character (which correlates with Carnival traditions) there are many pig stables and goat farmers at the locations of the Carnival. So, distribution does not even have to be via carnival gatherings. Most large floats are made and parked precisely IN the stables of farms, and the makers of them frolic everywhere through the mud and straw the day before, shake the farmer's hand and eat another sandwich there. Then embrace each other during parades and also the public along the way.

The south-eastern provinces of North Brabant and Limburg house over 63% of the country's 12 million pigs and 42% of its 101 million chickens. Intensive livestock production produces large amounts of ammonia. Concentrations are at highest in air samples from the south-east of the Netherlands.

Results in treatment of Covid-19 pneumonia

The coronavirus is a miniscule little nail bomb that is able to invade living body cells and take advantage of host cell protein synthesis and to produce offspring allowing hundreds of new virus particles to exit the host cell and spread throughout the body, resulting in a mortally ill patient. Several treating physicians have reported success in the treatment of patients with fever and COVID-19 pneumonia with Azithromycin. Azithromycin, a macrolide antibiotic, erythromycin and also doxycycline prevent viruses from multiplying by interfering with their protein synthesis in the host cell. It binds to the ribosomes in the host cell, inhibiting the transport of RNA and protein synthesis from viruses, preventing multiplication and spread in the body.

The majority of deaths in the 1918–1919 influenza pandemic likely resulted directly from secondary bacterial pneumonia caused by common upper respiratory-tract bacteria. Data from subsequent 1957 and 1968 pandemics are consistent with these findings. Antibiotics have also proven to favorably influence the course of the disease in pneumonia during these influenza epidemics. In the time of the 1918-1919 pandemic there was no antibiotic. Alexander Fleming discovered penicillin only in 1928.

Morens DM, Taubenberger JK, Fauci AS. Predominant Role of Bacterial Pneumonia as a Cause of Death in Pandemic Influenza: Implications for Pandemic Influenza Preparedness. J Infect Dis. 2008 Oct 1;198(7): 962–70

Patients with COVID-19 have been reported to be similarly at risk of secondary bacterial pneumonia, either as a consequence of damage inflicted by the novel coronavirus itself or invasive procedures such as intubation/mechanical ventilation to manage respiratory failure. Long-term immobilization in intensive care has also led to thrombosis and embolization.

Don't just take alone paracetamol with this rapidly progressing respiratory tract infection but also giving an adequate antibiotic such as azithromycin or doxycycline immediately with a fever can prevent worse.

Q fever epidemic

Manure and straw from the goats are distributed by farmers as fertilization over the land. Infected pregnant milk goats spread spores of the bacteria, after giving birth, with the afterbirth and amniotic fluid in the straw. As a result, the Coxiella-burnetii bacterium and spores spread through the air, infecting the local population in North Brabant, even after inhaling 100 germs.

In 2007 the first outbreak of Q fever in humans took place in the Netherlands. In Northeast Brabant, 73 patients with Q fever were observed around several dairy goat farms infected with *Coxiella burnetii*. In 2008, another epidemic of Q fever occurred in a wider area than in 2007. With 906 confirmed patients, this is the largest recorded Q fever epidemic in the world. In 2009 it became clear that the disease had spread over a large part of the Netherlands, almost 2,300 new infections were found. According to the official count up to March 2010, ten people have died of a chronic form of the disease. At the height of the Q fever outbreak in 2009-2010, ninety companies were infected. Infected animals can transmit Q fever to humans.

The bacteria end up in the environment because infected animals (which do not have to show any symptoms themselves) secrete bacteria. They do this through body fluids, such as tears, urine, mucus, saliva, milk and amniotic fluid. A lot of bacteria are released, especially during calving or lambing. Especially when it comes to an abortion. People are infected by inhaling contaminated dust particles. The severity of the infection depends on the number of germs inhaled. In the open air, the bacteria spread as a spore and can survive in this form for a long time. After inhalation, the bacteria can be absorbed into the bloodstream via the lungs and spread further in the body, with in some cases resulting in a chronic illness. The bacteria can only multiply in living cells. Q fever does not pass from person to person.

As with Q fever pneumonia and Chlamydia pneumonia, the long-term consequences of Covid pneumonia are insufficiently known. Will a smoker who has suffered from Covid pneumonia still have a greatly increased risk of lung cancer after a decade?

Lung cancer epidemic in The Netherlands, Belgium and UK

Country	Cigarette packs of 20 per year in 1970	Lung cancer mortality 1984 (CBS Netherlands) 2010 (EUROSTAT)	
Italy	84	77	73
Norway	88	43	71
France	92	65	87
Finland	93	87	73
Netherlands	**108**	**117**	**108**
Belgium	**119**	**119**	**115**
West Germany	125	73	West & East Germany 79
Japan	*141*	*43*	
United Kingdom	**153**	**100**	**82**
USA	*184*	*84*	

Age standardized lung cancer mortality (ICD 162 per 100,000 men per year) in ten different countries in 1984 and 2010 in relation to per adult consumption of manufactured / hand-rolled cigarettes in 1970.

- **In Japan and the USA has always been a lot more smoking and mortality rates of lung cancer were much lower.**

In 2012, cancer was the cause of 31% of all deaths in the Netherlands (Eurostat). Today about half of all men and one third of all women develop cancer and about 20% of all deaths are due to cancer. This is an impressive increase and seems to show that the increase in cancer is a recent biological event.

In 2019, 14,000 people developed lung cancer

Only 3,000 of these will be alive in 2024 (19% survival rate after five years). Lung cancer is not contagious but demands a lot from health care year after year. Every day 128 people die of cancer in the Netherlands. After diagnosed with colon cancer, the chance of being alive after five years is about 60%. For breast cancer, the chance of being alive five years after diagnosis is about 85%, much more favorable than for lung cancer.

Netherlands, Belgium and the United Kingdom have the highest lung cancer mortality of any country in Europe. Besides smoking, the hobby and breeding of tropical birds are the reason for this excess mortality.

- **More lung cancer in the Netherlands, Belgium and the United Kingdom. These three countries have the largest share in the international trade and import of tropical birds via Amsterdam Schiphol, Brussels Zaventem and London Heathrow respectively.**

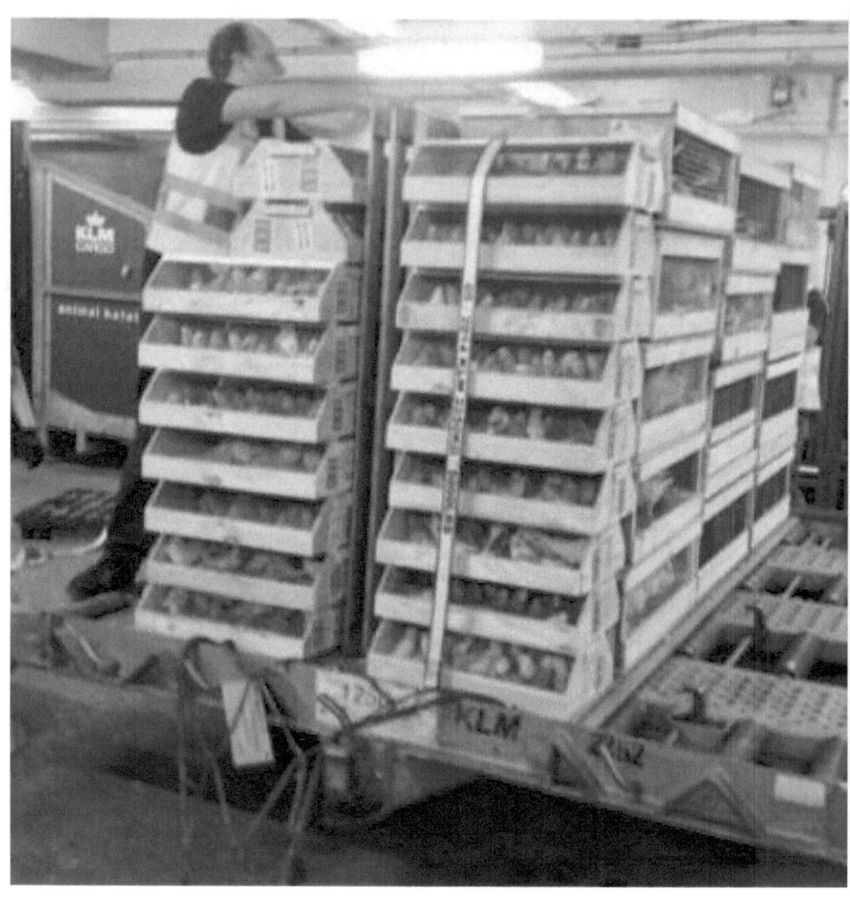

Transport of tropical birds via Amsterdam Schiphol

Bird exhibitions and bird breeders caused an explosive growth of this popular hobby

Since the slave trade and slavery were abolished 150 years ago, international trade in tropical companion animals, international human trafficking, the arms industry and drug trafficking became the most profitable forms of trade. Worldwide, an estimated 40,000 primates, 4 million exotic birds, 640,000 reptiles and 350 million tropical fish are traded live each year. The trade in exotics is estimated at an $ 6 billion industry.

My PhD research has shown that keeping and breeding tropical birds is mainly a hobby of young families. The ratio of breeders to the total number of bird keepers is about 1: 6. The level of organization of the large bird breeders in the Netherlands is greatly due to participation in the breeding competitions. Public shows, which were held several times a year, made the hobby increasingly popular in the twentieth century. When pigeons are kept together with tropical birds, Chlamydia infections are more common.

In the Netherlands were 7.5 million birds in households in 1984. The American Veterinary Medicine Association (AVMA) counted 11-16 million companion birds and exotic birds in the United States in 2007. In France, 6 million companion birds were owned by households in 2010. In Belgium every bred bird must be provided with a ring with a number to which the owner can identify the breeder. In 2011 the Association Ornithology de Belgique (AOB) registered 249 ornithological associations. Exotic birds such as larger parrots, macaw or cockatoo are traded legally or illegally from Asia or South America.

Tropical birds were late in history brought to the Old World. Increasingly larger numbers were taken as trophies by sailors, after the colonization of South America and the Caribbean. Only with the increase of shipping traffic and air cargo, tropical birds could easily be imported and traded in Europe. The largest epidemic of psittacosis occurred in 1929-1930 after the import of infected parrots from Argentina to Europe. Hundreds of people became seriously ill and 20% died after an acute fulminant disease. Initially, strict import restrictions were imposed in many countries. Not much later, parrots were again mass-imported.

Bird shows and bird breeders produced an explosive growth of this popular pastime. The housing of tropical birds in Western Europe has led to the adaptation of the psittacosis "virus", first in the flocks of the pigeon breeders who often kept also tropical birds. With many tropical bird breeders, the 'psittacosis virus' adapted and the disease that occurred in humans was less violent. The Chlamydia pneumoniae has adapted in Western Europe and the epidemic of bird flu (ornithosis) and Chlamydia pneumonia were the result of this. Chlamydia pneumonia is adjusted so that this microorganism now also passes from human to human through the airways and is now so prevalent in society that 98% have been infected. Repeated infections with Chlamydia, primarily occurring with bird breeders and bird keepers cause chronic respiratory diseases and cause lung cancer in humans.

From 1-4-1985 to 1-1-1987, 49 patients with lung cancer were under 65 in the study in hospitals in The Hague. Of these, 21 (43%) had small cell lung cancer. Of these patients, 14 (67%) had birds in the home 5-14 years before the diagnosis of small cell lung cancer. This form of lung cancer has the worst chance of survival. The survival rate after five years is only 8%.

Why so much lung cancer in North Brabant?

It is dangerous to smoke, but more dangerous in Belgium, the Netherlands and United Kingdom. Especially in the east of North Brabant in the surrounding of Tilburg it is most dangerous to smoke. Is this due to the carnival or is there more going on?

Organized bird breeders as at 1-1-1984 per province

North Brabant (male population 1.054.281) 23.009 (2.2%)
South Holland (1.539.994) 15.612 (1%)
Gelderland (859.840) 14.638 (1.7%)
Limburg (540.669) 12.426 (2.3%)
Overijssel (519.800) 10.096 (1.9%)
North Holland (1.123.305) 8.973 (0.8%)
Utrecht (454.452) 6.966 (1.5%)
Friesland (269.902) 5.223 (1.9%)
Zeeland (176.736) 5.046 (2.9%)
Groningen (278.747) 4.952 (1.8%)
Drenthe (213.472) 3.726 (1.7%)
The Netherlands (male population 7.067.198) 110.667 (1.6%)

Most of the bird clubs and organized birdkeepers are found in Limburg and North Brabant, above all in Tilburg. The number of organized bird breeders of the Netherlands society of bird lovers grew from 1.400 in the year 1940 to 45.800 in 1984.

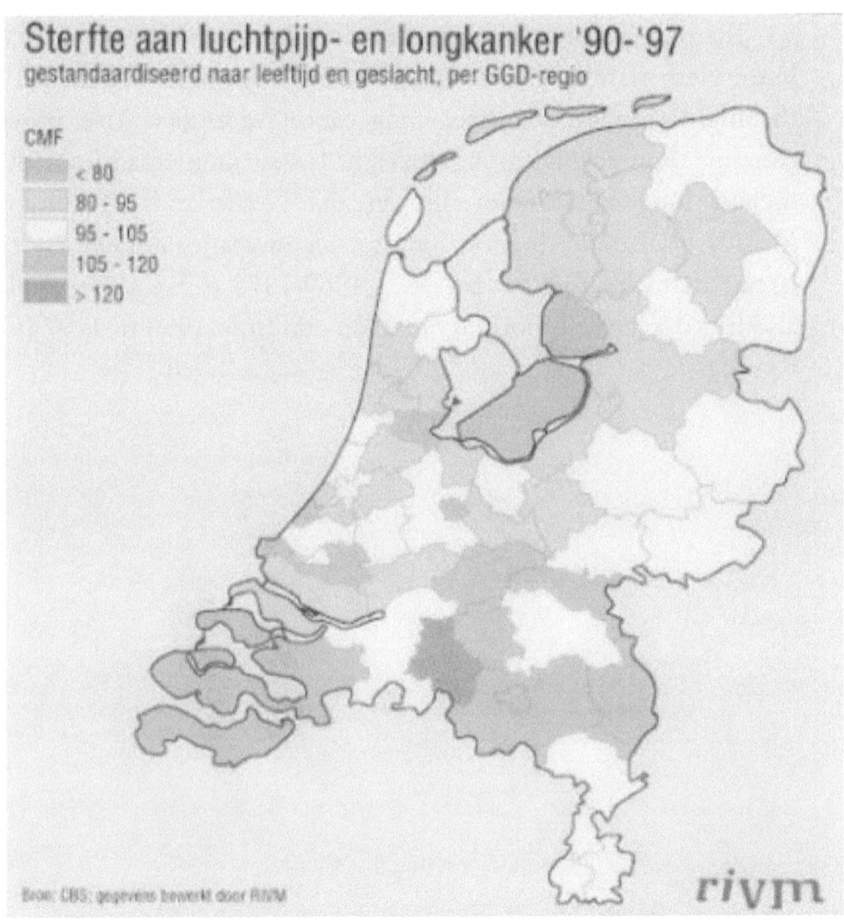

- *Since 1969, the province of North Brabant had the highest age-standardized lung cancer mortality.*
- *Most of the bird clubs and organized birdkeepers are traditionally found in this province, above all in Tilburg.*
- *Also from 1990 until 1997 North Brabant had the highest lung cancer mortality in the Netherlands and again Tilburg.*

There are regional differences in mortality from lung cancer in men in the Netherlands. The rural province of North Brabant had, in 1984, the highest age-standardized lung cancer mortality. This province contains three towns among the eight largest municipalities with the highest lung cancer mortality in the Netherlands. Tilburg and Maastricht had the highest lung cancer mortality among the eight largest municipalities for the years 1969-1978 (CBS 1980). Tilburg also had the highest mortality in 1984 and from 1990 to 1997 (CBS, RIVM).

Lung cancer mortality (per 100000 men per year) in different Dutch provinces and large municipalities

		1969 -1978	1984
North Brabant		91	114
	Tilburg	**117**	**131**
	Eindhoven	98	121
	Breda	98	117
Utrecht		89	109
Limburg		93	104
	Maastricht	103	92
Overijssel		75	104
North-Holland		95	104
	Haarlem	11	114
	Amsterdam	100	104
South-Holland		92	103
	Rotterdam	102	123
	Leiden	99	102
Gelderland		77	102
Groningen		67	90
Friesland		62	89
Drenthe		60	88
Zeeland		60	86

From 1990 until 1997 North Brabant had again the highest lung cancer mortality in the Netherlands and again Tilburg.

The incidence of lung cancer was quite low in the Netherlands until 1950. In 1950, 1.179 men and 167 women died from this disease. By 1983, the numbers had increased to 7.104 men and 800 women.

Chlamydia pneumonia (Cpn) causes lung cancer

Long-term studies using cigarette smoking machines, in hamsters, dogs and monkeys, did not show a statistically significant increase in malignant tumors in the airways, although very long exposures and high doses of smoke were used (Coggins CR 2001). These inhalation studies were performed without additional respiratory infection of the test animals. The tobacco industry has long cited the studies as evidence of no increase in lung cancer from smoking.

An animal model for lung cancer was developed by repeated injection of Chlamydia pneumonia bacteria into rat airways, with or without the most carcinogenic component of the cigarette benzo (a) pyrene (**Chu DJ 2012**). With the combination of benzo (a) pyrene and the bacteria of tropical bird flu in the spray, 44% of the laboratory rats developed lung cancer. The combined factors of smoking and chronic Cpn infection have effects on each other and lead to a greatly increased risk of lung cancer.

Chu DJ, Guo SG, Pan CF, Wang J, Du Y, Lu XF, Yu ZY (2012) An experimental model for induction of lung cancer in rats by Chlamydia pneumoniae. Asian Pac J Cancer Prev. 2012; 13 (6): 2819-22

Favorable results of combined therapy of azithromycin with the chemotherapy on non-small cell lung cancer patients

Although new chemotherapeutic drugs have been applied constantly, their efficacy for non-small cell lung cancer (NSCLC) is still not satisfactory.

In recent years, epidemiological investigations have shown that lung cancer may be induced by chronic Chlamydia pneumonia (Cpn) infection. This study (Chu DJ 2014) of azithromycin, commonly used for the treatment of Cp infections, combined with the chemotherapeutics paclitaxe and cisplatin on stage III-IV NSCLC patients achieved favorable results in terms of side effects and overall survival.

How are infections related to lung cancer?

Smallest bacteria as Chlamydia and retroviruses are related to the development of lung cancer. Half of the biomass on earth exists of monomers. Unicellular organisms such as bacteria, yeast cells, amoebae and viruses divide themselves interminable. Tumor cell lines share this property. Multi-cellular organisms have this property only in their stem cells and germ cells. All other cells die after about 50 cell divisions.

Of the unicellular organisms, smallest spore forming bacteria as Chlamydia and viruses are obligate cell parasites. They are the most successful and efficient in reproduction of their genome (Clark 1996). That detracts nothing from the fact that they first need to infect a living cell. When Chlamydia enter bronchus epithelial cells they remain latent and persistent. When they integrate in the genome of the basal epithelial cell they could lead to the development of a tumor cell. After about 30 tumor cell divisions there is a discernible tumor. These processes take at least 10-15 years.

Chlamydia pneumoniae was found to be serologically associated with lung cancer (Laurila 1997; Koyi 1999; Jackson 2000)

Laurila et al. found chronic Chlamydia pneumoniae infection in 52% of lung cancer patients (n=230) and in 45% of controls. The incidence was especially increased in men younger than 60 years (3 times more often than in the controls) but not in men over 60 years old.

Jackson et al. also found an increased risk of lung cancer in subjects younger than 60 years of age with previous Chlamydia pneumoniae infection, but not in older subjects.

N.B. Rearing tropical birds is mainly a hobby of young families.

Results for treatment of malignant lymphomas

Malignant lymphomas were treated with tetracycline (doxycycline) and their disappearance was accompanied by the eradication of the Chlamydia pneumonia bacteria detected in the cells (**Ferreri AJ 2006**). Chlamydia psittaci (Cp), the bacterium of psittacose has often been shown in malignant lymphomas. The bacterium has been shown in the tumor tissue, taken out and cell cultures are made. By treatment with doxycycline (tetracycline) malignant lymphomas are cured **(Ferreri AJ 2012**). Treatment with doxycycline (twice daily 100 mg) for six months disappeared the malignant lymphomas in 64% of patients.

The Chlamydia bacterium has no cell wall and, like viruses, is completely dependent on mucous membrane cells in the airways. By entering a body cell, the bacteria come to life. Then it will copy itself. In the end, hundreds of new bacteria leave the cell and spread further into the airways and body. Once in the host cell, Chlamydia is not sensitive to penicillin. Tetracycline enters in contaminated body cells by diffusion along membrane pores. Once in the cell, tetracyclines and doxycycline inhibit internal cell metabolism, DNA and protein synthesis, preventing the Chlamydia cell parasites from producing new proteins for growth and multiplication.

Indoor Air Pollution

Significantly increased dust levels are measured in households where birds are kept. Particulate matter with a diameter of 2.5 micron or less is the most important health risk of (indoor) air pollution. The number of particles of about 2 microns is increased in bird-keeping households. Due to excessive mucus production, there is more drainage of alveoli in smokers than in non-smokers. As a result, the dust and antigen load are shifted from the alveoli to the smaller air tubes in the bird keeper who smokes.

- **The smaller bronchi are the preferred location of lung cancer**

Both smoking and keeping birds are ultimately responsible for the poor functioning of the "lung cleaning service" and a shortage of immune proteins. The result is less protection of the lung mucosal cells against continual allergen and fine material that precipitates on the thin mucus layer of the smaller air tubes. Most lung tumors develop in the smaller air tubes, at some distance from the alveoli, where gases and dust particles circulate at first instance.

The impact of air pollution on health.

Smog can carry large amounts of poisonous and harmful substances and penetrate deep into the lungs and blood circulation through the respiratory tract, thereby affecting human health. The Global Burden of Disease Study 2010 ranked particulate matter as the 8th highest cause of death worldwide, when considering estimated deaths attributable to the independent effects of 67 risk factors. In China, this ranking could be as high as 4th, accounting for approximately 1.2 million premature deaths in 2010. The Big Smog of 1952 in London caused about 12,000 deaths in five days. Coal fired in stoves and factories was the cause.

PM2.5, which is defined as fine particulate matter with an aerodynamic diameter of 2.5 micrometers or less, is the main health hazard of smog.

PM 2.5 penetrate deeply into the lungs through the respiratory tract due to its small size and irritate and corrode the alveolar wall. The resulting impaired lung function would show as coughs, wheezes, respiratory disorders and other symptoms, and increase the risks of bronchial asthma, chronic obstructive pulmonary disease (COPD), emphysema and other respiratory diseases.

Huge increase in meat production in the West

The increase in meat products and dairy production in the West could only be achieved with artificial insemination of mammals and the animals unilaterally fattening with soy flour, corn and fish meal.

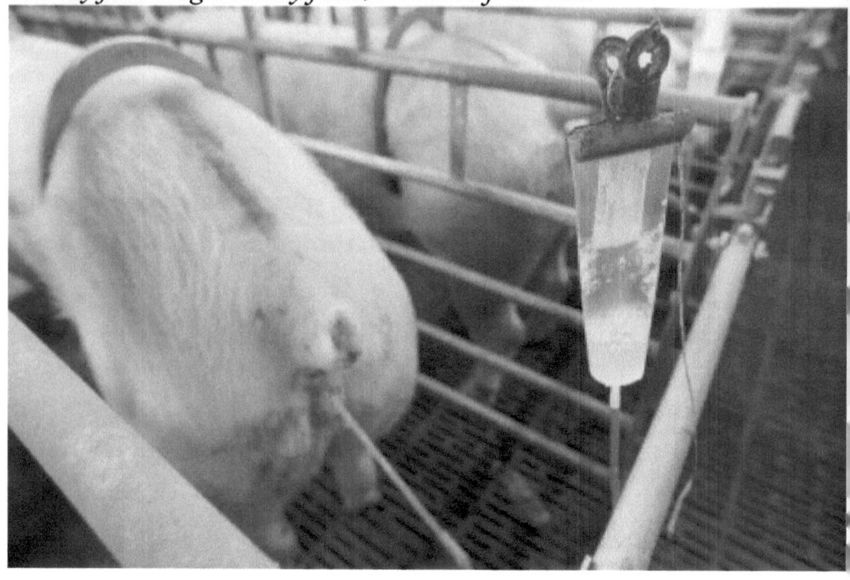

Artificial insemination of pigs in a factory farm

- Unbridled breeding of animals, through artificial insemination of cattle and with incubators for poultry, has a devastating effect on our health, nature and the climate.
- Fast food, unnatural food and meat consumption lead to obesity, vitamin deficiencies, chronic diseases and premature death.
- Cancer is now the main cause of premature death.

Slaughter Animals	
	Pigs
	Weaning pigs
	Rabbits
	Dairy cows
	Calves
	Milk goats
	Lambs
	Laying hens
	Broiler chickens
	Civets
	Minks
	Bats
	Mountain marmots
	Chimpanzees
	Dromedaries
	Wildlife
	Whales

Humans take up all the space on earth, most slaughter animals are artificially fertilized and fattened in stables or cages.

Before 1950, the bull runner would visit farms to fertilize the cow.

What are the risks of higher meat production?

An increased mortality of brain tumors has been observed in veterinary surgeons (Blair A). Veterinarians and Artificial Insemination assistants do a lot of internal research on cows. Transmission of the bovine leukemia virus (BLV) via the uterus and the birth canal during labor, plays a crucial role in the spread and persistence of BLV infection in cattle.

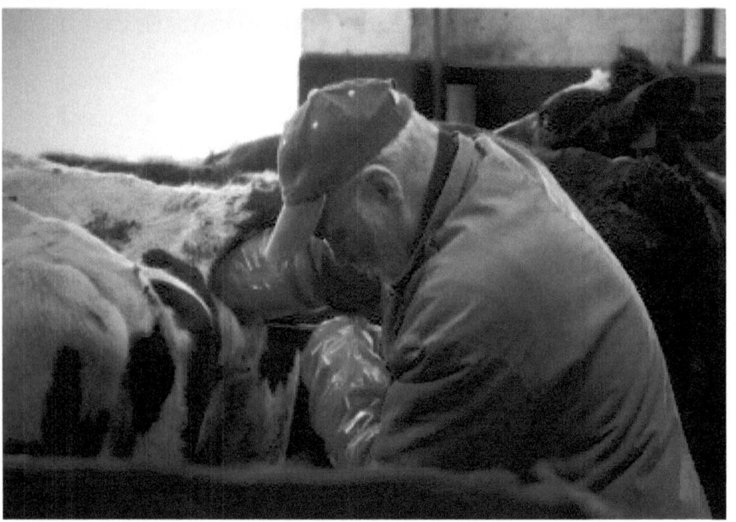

In their work, veterinarians and AI staff come into contact with bovine leukemia virus (BLV), a carcinogenic virus. Bovine leukemia is an economically important infection of dairy cattle worldwide.

The presence of infections in Canadian dairy herds is high and is still increasing. Seventy percent of the herds were identified as BLV positive (one or more positive animals).

Nekouei O, VanLeeuwen J, Sanchez J, Kelton D, Tiwari A, Keefe G Herd-level risk factors for infection with bovine leukemia virus in Canadian dairy herds. Prev Vet Med. 2015; 119 (3-4)

The deaths of 5,016 veterinarians were examined and compared with those of the general American population. The mortality rates were significantly increased from malignant lymphomas and leukemia, colon, brain and skin. Less mortality was found for stomach and lung cancer.

Blair A, Hayes HM Jr. (1982) Mortality patterns among US veterinarians, 1947-1977: an expanded study. Int J Epidemiol. 1982 Dec;11(4):391-7.

Increased risk of esophageal, colon, brain and pancreatic cancer and melanoma in veterinarians in Sweden could not be explained by the socio-economic status of this profession. Occupational exposures to carcinogenic viruses in livestock are potential sources.

Travier N, Gridley G, Blair A, Dosemeci M, Boffetta P. Cancer incidence among male Swedish veterinarians and other workers of the veterinary industry: a record-linkage study. Cancer Causes Control. 2003 (6):587-93.

Cows are constantly re-impregnated after the birth of the calves by artificial insemination, so that their milk will never stop flowing.

Artificial insemination (AI) in cows was introduced in Friesland in 1935.The semen of the bull is frozen in "straws" and then introduced into the animal by a veterinarian or AI assistant. Calves are taken away from their mother soon after birth.

Their calves grow up to become dairy cows or are reared for veal. For production of milk and cheese, the mother cow must give birth to as many calves as possible. Milk, cheese and meat production are inextricably linked.

Raw egg proteins and raw milk products

Industrially processed food contains a large proportion of liquid chicken egg proteins that in some cases are not sufficiently heated processed. Eggs are beaten on crushers, yolk and whites are separated, eggshells and hail strings are removed through filters and the protein product is heated to 56 ° Celsius.

In the Netherlands (1983), 20,000 tons of liquid chicken protein was produced for the industry, marginally pasteurized sometimes insufficiently heat treated. The confectioner processes a large number of products that contain eggs. This can be the pasteurized proteins, or he processes fresh eggs. The "whites" are collected in a special container. Housewives also sometimes come into contact with raw egg proteins when making cake batter or desserts at home. Or if they whip up the raw egg proteins.

Raw egg proteins are processed in:

SUGAR GLAZE raw egg whites with powdered sugar

ROOM FONDANT raw egg whites with butter, sugar and liqueur

OMELET SIBÉRIEN raw egg whites with sugar

BAVAROIS raw egg whites with sugar, cream, gelatin, fruits

ICE CREAM raw egg whites with sugar, milk and cream.

And in:

STEAK TARTAR with a raw egg

Raw milk products

Raw milk is milk from cows, sheep, or goats that has not been pasteurized to kill harmful bacteria and viruses. Raw milk and cheese made from raw milk also contain raw proteins and can harbor harmful bacteria and viruses.

Employees risks in the poultry industry

Carcinogenic viruses are found and cause tumors in chickens and turkeys. A number are carriers and diffusers of these viruses. Virus has been shown in chicken products and eggs, so exposure to humans is universal and almost unavoidable. These viruses are not very contagious, but still have the ability to infect and transform human cells. Antibodies against avian leukemia viruses (ALV) and Reticulo Endothelial Viruses (REV) have been found in blood sera of workers in poultry slaughterhouses. Mortality from cancer has been studied in 20,132 workers in poultry slaughterhouses and processing plants, a group with the highest human exposure to these viruses. Substantially increased risks were observed in poultry workers as a whole or in subgroups, for different cancers: cancer of the mouth and pharynx; pancreas; trachea / bronchus / lung; brain; cervix; lymphocytic leukemia; monocytic leukemia; and tumors of the blood-forming and lymphatic systems.

Metayer C, Johnson ES, Rice JC (1998) Nested case-control study of tumors of the hemopoietic and lymphatic systems among workers in the meat industry. Am J Epidemiol 147(8):727-38

Johnson ES, Ndetan H, Lo KM (2010) Cancer mortality in poultry slaughtering / processing plant workers belonging a union pension fund. Environ Res 110(6):588-94

Brain cancer is more common in poultry farmers involved in killing chickens. The killing of chickens was accompanied by an almost 6-fold increase in the risk of brain cancer. Workers in poultry slaughterhouses and processing plants often process thousands of chickens daily, come into contact with poultry meat, organs and blood and run the risk of injuries that form a route for viruses and other microbial substances to enter the body. They also work for longer periods in confined spaces, which increases the risk of inhaling microbes. Viruses that are known to cause cancer in poultry can be responsible for the increased incidence of cancer in poultry farmers killing chickens.

Gandhi S, Felini MJ, Nidetan H, Cardarelli K, Jadhav S, Faramawi M, **Johnson ES** (2014) A pilot case cohort study of brain cancer in poultry and control workers. Nutr Cancer.

Professor E.S. Johnson, an epidemiologist at the University of Fort Worth Texas, has developed and patented the only test to date that can detect the presence of carcinogenic viruses in the genome of tumor cells of workers with these cancers.

How are animals in megafarms fed?

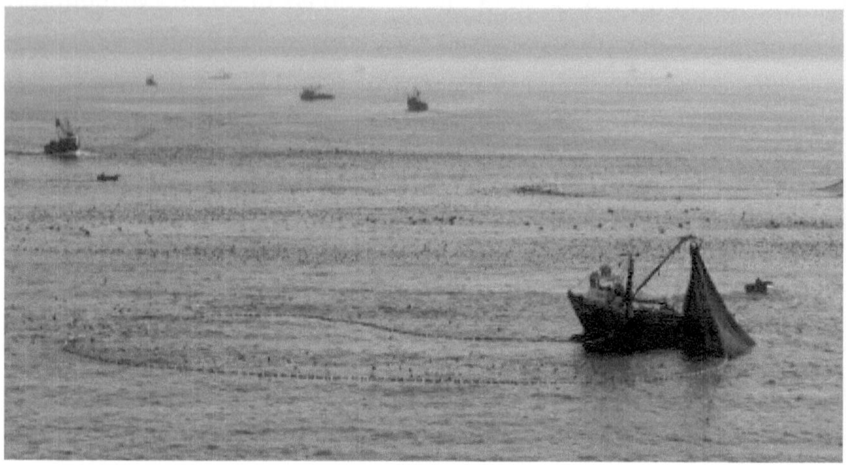

Anchovy from the southeast of the Pacific Ocean is sold as cattle feed to Europe's factory farms. Approximately one third of the total catch is fed to consumption animals, mostly farmed fish, pigs and chickens. European fishermen are obliged to land all by-catches by 2020. In addition to the by-catches, the fish-processing industry also produces a significant amount of reusable waste, such as skins, bones, fish heads and internal organs. Fish meal can be created by hydrolysis of the fish from the by-catches and fish remains, which is a great need. Especially at the fish farms in the Mediterranean.

Tuna, salmon, cattle, pigs and chickens grow faster and fatter by fishmeal. More profit can be achieved and the time to slaughter is shortened. For production of fish oil and fishmeal, some 20-30 million tons of fish, anchovies, herring, mackerel and sprat species have been removed from the southeastern Pacific Ocean over the past decades.

Going back 1000 years in Europe, it was declines in freshwater fish thanks to human pressure which first pushed fishermen out into the oceans in larger numbers. Five hundred years ago, it was the decline of coastal fish that brought deep-sea trawling into existence. Worldwide 20 billion is awarded annually. 6.3 billion is spent on subsidies for fuel alone; an extra 8 billion goes to the maintenance of the major ports.

Small fishing uses 75% less energy to catch the same volume of fish, more environmentally friendly and with many more people.

Mega farms with only cows, calves, pigs or chickens feed the animals with soy flour, fish meal and low doses of antibiotics to fatten the animals faster and to gain more profit. This has drastically increased the animal fat content of steak, pork and chicken meat.

Diseases in later life by consuming fast food

Increased consumption of energy, animal proteins, animal fats and red meat was produced in different regions of the world after the transition to a more industrialized diet, hamburgers, sugary drinks and fast food in these countries. With more than 225 million overweight people in 2016, the USA has the largest number of overweight people in the world. The USA also export these unhealthy eating habits around the world. Worse diet is the leading cause of morbidity and mortality in the United States. With an average life expectancy of 78.1 years the United States comes in only at number fifty of the world ranking list, despite being the richest nation on the planet with the most advanced medical technology. The Netherlands is slightly better with an average life expectancy of 79.2 years, less than most other European countries. Even in spite of the nation's alarming high suicide rate Japanese live 82.1 years on average.

Diseases relating to diet are the leading causes of death to the United States, even surpassing smoking.

The number of overweight or obese people increased between 1990 and 2016. Poor diet contributed to 14 percent, while smoking accounted for 11 percent. Obesity and high blood pressure accounted for 11 and 8 percent respectively. The number one cause of death in America is the American diet.

When people move from low- to high-risk countries, their disease rates almost always change to those of the new environment. New diet, new diseases. But the reverse is also true. If we're eating the Standard American Diet and switch to a diet higher in whole plant foods, such as fruits and vegetables, this may lower your risk.

Cancer is now the most common cause of death in Western Europe, more often than chronic obstructive pulmonary disease (COPD) and cardiovascular disease and diabetes (IHD). While mortality rates for COPD and IHD are declining due to improved health care, mortality rates for cancer have increased. Consumption of animal fats and proteins has increased considerably since the last century. The production of meat (products), poultry, pork and other meat tripled between 1980 and 2010 and is likely to double again by 2050. At present, 70 billion farm animals are being bred annually for food.

As we get older, we notice which unhealthy lifestyle habits have taken possession of us. The body constantly renews itself through the ingested diet and within a few years all cells and tissues are constantly being completely rebuilt. With age, the choice of animal or vegetable protein and fat in the daily diet is of great importance for protection against chronic diseases and cancer. Cardiovascular disease, obesity and uncontrolled growth of derailed cells are the result of an excess of animal proteins and fats in the daily diet. The chicken leukemia virus and bovine leukemia virus in our food chain are related to common cancers. The time without symptoms is 50% - 70% of the total growth of a tumor and cancer usually reveals itself at a later age.

In Japan and Korea, large-scale imports of beef and pork began after the Second World War, respectively after the Korean War. In 1970 in Japan and 1990 in Korea a sharp increase in the numbers of colon cancer was observed. Consumption of fried beef (eg shabu-shabu, Korean yukhoe and Japanese yukke) became very popular in both countries.

A specific meat factor, presumably one or more thermo-resistant carcinogenic bovine viruses (for example polyoma, papilloma or single-stranded DNA viruses), can contaminate the beef and lead to latent infections in the intestinal tract.

Zur Hausen H (2012) Red meat consumption and cancer: reasons for suspect involvement or bovine infectious factors in colorectal cancer. Int J Cancer. 2012 Jun 1; 130 (11): 2475-83

Increased consumption of energy, animal fat and Red meat has occurred in East Asia in recent decades. Data on breast cancer, colon, prostate, esophagus and stomach cancer mortality rates for China (1988-2000), Hong Kong (1960-2006), Japan (1950-2006), Korea (1985-2006) and Singapore (1963- 2006) were obtained from the WHO. In the selected countries (except breast cancer in Hong Kong), a noticeable increase in mortality rates of breast, colon and prostate cancer and a decrease in esophageal and gastric cancer in the study periods were observed. For example, the annual percentage increase in mortality in breast cancer was 5.5% for the period 1985-1993 in Korea and the mortality rates for prostate cancer increased from 1958 to 1993 in Japan by 3.2% per year.

These changes in cancer mortality followed about 10 years after the transition to more industrially prepared food, hamburgers, sugary drinks and fast food in these countries.

Zhang J, Dhakai IB, Zhao Z, Li L (2012) Trends in mortality from cancers of the breast, colon, prostate, esophagus, and stomach in East Asia: role of nutrition transition. Eur J Cancer Prev 2012 Sep; 21 (5): 480-9

Mortality rates for prostate cancer have increased dramatically (25x) in Japan after the Second World War. After the war the consumption of milk increased by 20x, from meat 9x and from eggs 7x. Milk contains large amounts of estrogens plus proteins and saturated fats. The recent increase in its use is likely to be the cause of the surge of prostate cancer in Japan.

Ganmaa D, Li XM, Qin LQ et al. The experience of Japan as a clue to the etiology of testicular and prostatic cancers. Med Hypotheses. 2003 May; 60 (5): 724-30

The inhabitants of Tuvalu, Fiji, Samoa and the Cook Islands are massively overweight. According to the World Health Organization (WHO), nine of the world's ten thickest countries belong to the Pacific Islands. Tonga (4th, 90.8%), Samoa (6th, 80.4%) and USA (9th, 74.1%). Up to 95 percent of the adult population is overweight in some countries. The number of people with obesity, extremely overweight, varies from 35 to 50 percent.

The Cook Islands (90.9% overweight) are in third place in the world ranking. Slightly more than half of the population suffers from obesity. Inexpensive factory processed food has replaced the original diet of fresh fish and vegetables. Fresh fish is relatively expensive, with this money you can buy multiple hamburger meals. A bottle of cola is cheaper here than a bottle of water. 75% of the people on Samoa are extremely overweight.

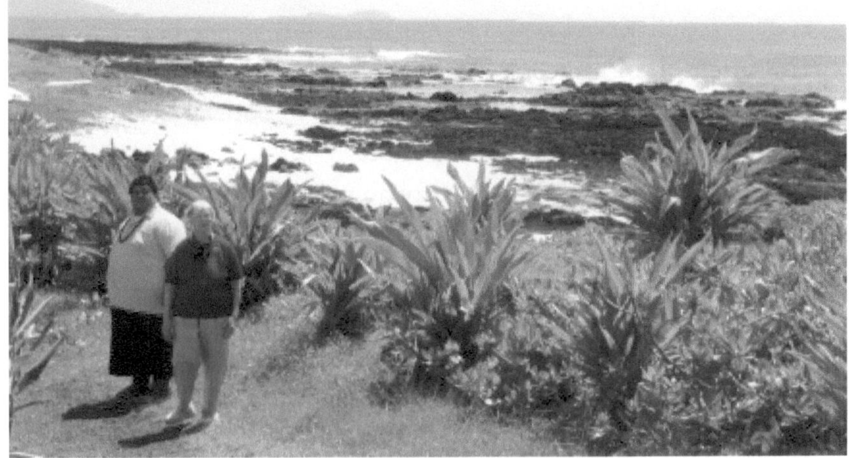

Recent increase in cancer

Bowel Cancer

An increased risk of colorectal cancer has long been shown for the consumption of undercooked red meat. In Japan and Korea, beef and pork were imported on a large scale after the Second World War and the Korean War. A strong increase in the number of patients with colon cancer was observed after 1970 in Japan and after 1990 in Korea. The consumption of undercooked beef (eg, Shabu-shabu, Korean Yukhoe and Japanese Yukke) became very popular in both countries.

Virus as a source of colon cancer

A specific beef factor, probably one or more heat-resistant carcinogenic bovine viruses (DNA-virus: for example, polyoma, papilloma and RNA-virus: bovine leukemia virus BLV) can infect the beef and cause latent and persistent intestinal infections after human consumption (**Zur Hausen H 2012**).

Polyoma viruses in hamburgers

In chopped beef samples three types of polyoma virus have been shown, which are resistant to BBQ temperatures and are carcinogenic to their natural hosts. The papilloma and polyoma viruses in particular are resistant to medium-heated steak tartar, in which central parts of the meat are not heated above 40 - 70 degrees Celsius. These viruses endure 80 degrees Celsius for 30 minutes without losing their ability to cause infections. These viruses are also insufficiently inactivated during the pasteurization of dairy products (Peretti A. 2015).

Acid-resistant bacteria and stomach cancer

Two Australian GPs realized that acid-solid bacteria can survive the acidic environment of the stomach, which other pathogenic bacteria cannot. They discovered Helicobacter pylori, which are causing severe stomach inflammatory disease. It was then discovered that these microbes cause gastric carcinoma.

Lichtman MA A Bacterial Cause of Cancer: An Historical Essay.
Oncologist. 2017 May;22(5):542-548

Zhang J, Dhakai IB, Zhao Z, Li L Trends in mortality from cancers of the breast, colon, prostate, oesophagus, and stomach in East Asia: role of nutrition transition. Eur J Cancer Prev 2012 Sep;21(5):480-9

Zur Hausen H (2012) Red meat consumption and cancer: reasons to suspect involvement of bovine infectious factors in colorectal cancer.
Int J Cancer.130(11):2475-83

Breast Cancer

People are exposed to carcinogenic viruses that often occur in animals in the food chain, such as laying hens, eggs, broiler chickens and dairy cows. The Avian Leukemia Virus (ALV) and Bovine Leukemia Viruses (BLV) are RNA viruses and have been shown in breast cancer cells.

Bovine Leukemia Virus (BLV) has been shown in breast cancer cells

Breast cancer and ovarian cancer were rare in Japan, compared with other countries. The mortality rates, however, are increasing. After the Second World War changes in lifestyle took place in Japan. In the years 1947-1997, mortality rates of breast and ovarian cancer increased 2- and 4-fold, and the respective intake of milk, meat and eggs increased 20, 10 and 7-fold. The increase in death rates from breast cancer and ovarian cancer could be attributed to increased consumption of animal nutrition, which occurred after 1945.

Milk, dairy products and eggs are probably the cause of this (Buehring). Cows are often infected with bovine leukemia virus (BLV), a carcinogenic virus that can be transferred from the cow to the calf via the milk or during birth. Most infected cattle seem healthy and the infection is persistent. Consumption of non-pasteurized dairy products, or cheese made from raw milk, or insufficiently heated beef at the BBQ can transmit this infectious virus to humans. About 38% of the cattle, 84% of the dairy herd, and 100% of factory farm herds in the US are infected with BLV. Less than 5% of these cattle get leukemia. With this condition the animals are not admitted to the US consumer market.

The BLV virus circulates with the white blood cells through the blood of infected cattle. The BLV virus also infects the mammary gland cells of the cows and infected cells are found in cow's milk (Lanou AJ). Pasteurization of cow's milk makes the BLV ineffective.

Buehring GC (2015) has shown that 39% of people in a San Francisco Bay Area have antibodies against BLV in the blood, which is an indication of exposure to BLV. Almost all cow's milk contains BLV bovine leukemia virus. In a study of 213 women, BLV-related DNA was found in breast tissue of women with a diagnosis of breast cancer, not in breast tissue of women without history of breast cancer (Buehring GC 2014).

Ovarian and fallopian tube cancer in laying hens

Ovarian cancer often occurs in laying hens (Frederickson TN). For this reason, they are usually slaughtered after the first leg year. In poultry farms, laying hens do not become older than 24 months. Avian Leukemia Virus (leucosis) is a retrovirus that infects large parts of the modern poultry farms and caused a lot of economic damage. The virus is present in chickens and eggs. Man is exposed to this. RNA viruses are single-stranded proteins that do not accurately divide. When RNA viruses divide within a host cell, they make many copies that differ from the original. Some of these copy differences increase their genetic variation and survival chances in the host. Therefore, although it is often possible to prevent a DNA virus infection with a sustainable vaccine, it is very difficult, if not impossible, to make a sustainable vaccine for an RNA virus, especially the RNA retroviruses. This also makes RNA viruses very difficult to treat with medicines.

Mice also infect the grain stocks with a virus that is closely related to breast cancer viruses (Stewart TH). Free-range chickens are often outside, so that the risk of contamination due to the contamination of food on the ground by mouse droppings is greater.

In the winter months, mice often go to poultry farms to look for food. Virus spreading mice; contamination of cereals, chicken feeds and poultry; transfer by infected chickens from viruses to the eggs; processing of raw, insufficiently heated protein in confectionery products; this is how the ALV virus arrives in humans (Pham TD).

Raw proteins often contain leukemia virus (ALV and BLV)

Breast and colon cancer are not caused by breathing bad air. A causal relationship will be found earlier for pathogens in our diet. Animal proteins in milk and dairy products, in meat products and in egg proteins carry carcinogenic viruses. Improved laboratory techniques provide increasing evidence. A total of 22,788 persons with lactose intolerance were examined, who did not use milk products, and compared with people who did use milk products. The risk of lung, breast and colon cancer appeared to be significantly reduced in the group that did not use milk products. The risk of lung, breast and colon cancer appeared to be significantly reduced in the group that did not use milk products.

Ji J, Sundquist J, Sundquist K Lactose intolerance and reduced risk of lung, breast and ovarian cancers: aetiological clues from a population-based study in Sweden. Br J Cancer. 2015 Jan 6; 112 (1): 149-52

Breast cancer and ovarian cancer are they Zoonoses?

The observation that chickens may be infected with a closely related form of mouse breast cancer virus (MMTV) may be of epidemiological significance for human breast cancer. Chickens and eggs can be infected by mice and in turn pass the virus on to people. The successful infection of human cells by MMTV has already been demonstrated (Indik S 2007). MMTV can infect human cell cultures and this finding provides a possible explanation for the discovery of MMTV in patients with breast cancer. The numbers of breast cancer that occur in humans vary geographically. No environmental factor could explain this variation. The highest incidence of breast cancer worldwide occurs in countries where Mus domesticus is the native or imported type of house mouse.

Stewart TH, Sage RD, Stewart AF, Cameron DW (2000) Breast cancer incidence highest in the range of one species of house mouse, Mus domesticus. Br J Cancer. 82(2):446-51

Breast stem cells

Women who have remained childless have immature mammary cells with stem cell activity. When these cells become infected with carcinogenic virus, this infection leads to uncontrolled cell division.

In the twentieth century, breast cancer was also called "the nuns disease." Full-term pregnancies reduce the risk of breast cancer and the higher the number of pregnancies, the greater this protection. The risk of breast cancer decreases by 7% after every full-term pregnancy. Women who have given birth to children have a 30% lower risk than childless women. Breast cancer is most common in childless women and women around menopause. The biological regression of women begins around the time of menopause and is accompanied by a reduction of immune function of body cells. Reduced cell defenses can lead to the proliferation of infected mammary cells.

How great is the loss of animal and plant species?

- In the last 50 years homo sapiens has wiped out 60% of mammals, birds, fish and reptiles in the wild
- Humankind has destroyed 83% of all mammals and half of plants since the dawn of civilization.
- Wildlife hunting in tropical forests reduces bird and mammal populations.

Our ancestors have likely consumed bushmeat, wild animals killed for food. During the 20th century, however, commercial hunting using firearms and wire snares to supply logging and oil exploration concessions along new roadway networks has dramatically increased the catch in Central African forests. Annually, it is estimated that 579 million wild animals are caught and consumed in the Congo basin, equaling 4.5 million tons of meat, with the addition of a possible 5 million tons of wild mammalian meat from the Amazon basin. Tropical lowland forest habitat contains the world's greatest terrestrial biodiversity and may therefore harbor a reservoir of zoonotic pathogens.

The wildlife trade in general generates in excess one billion direct and indirect contacts between humans and domesticated animals annually. The broad range of tissue and fluid exposures associated with the bush meat industry's hunting and butchering may take these wildlife interactions especially risky. In Africa, as many as 30 different species of primates are hunted and processed by the bushmeat industry.

- One billion people suffer from hunger, while 70 billion animals are fattened and eaten every year.

We can no longer ignore the impact of current unsustainable production models.

Benítez-López A, Alkemade R, Schipper AM et al. The impact of hunting on tropical mammal and bird populations. Science 2017 356(6334):180-183

Population growth to seven, eight or nine billion causes food shortages, diseases and climate changes due to intensive meat production. The large number of animals locked up for meat consumption is the perfect system as a source for pathogenic viruses such as highly pathogenic influenza, corona virus and leukemia virus. The human race is moving in the same direction as the species that we have seen disappearing.

How do we make a greenhouse of the earth?

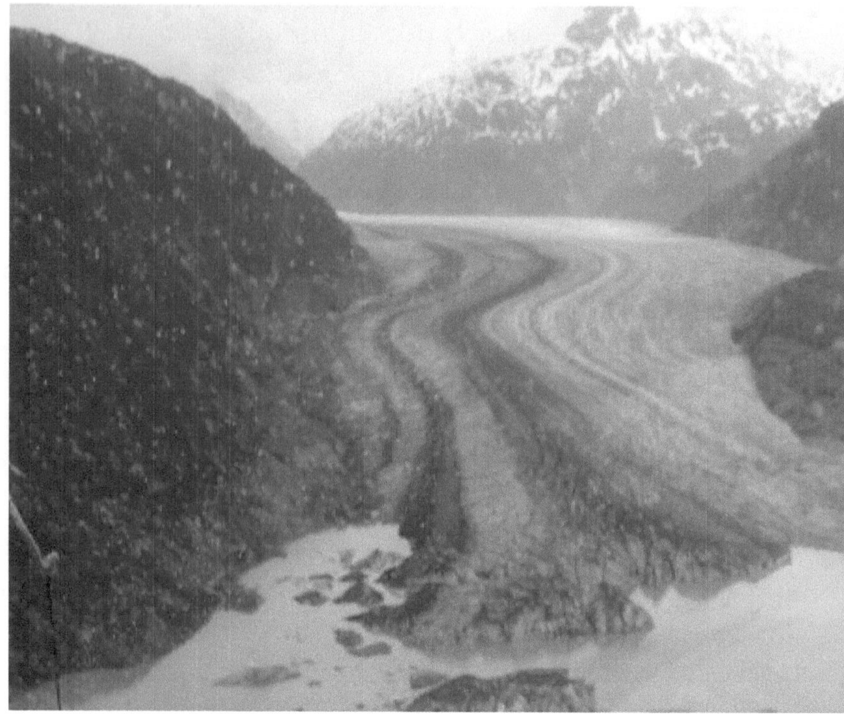

- Every year the glaciers in Alaska become hundreds of meters shorter by melting the ice.
- In the USA, cattle emit approximately 5.5 million m3 of methane, a greenhouse 25 times more potent than CO2.

Livestock farming accounts for at least 14.5% and, according to some studies, even 51% of man-made greenhouse gases.

CE Delft, Fraunhofer Institute for Systems and Innovation Research and LEI Wageningen. Behavioural climate change mitigation options and their appropriate inclusion in quantitative longer-term policy scenarios. Delft, January 2012

All life depends on the oceans. Circulation in the North Atlantic has slowed to the lowest level in centuries. The slowdown of the Gulf Stream devastates fisheries and will lead to a rise in sea levels. Large amounts of nitrogen from fertilizer and manure are distributed annually over agricultural land. No doubt that it increases crop yield, but plants do not absorb it completely, so that more fertilizer and animal waste is added than the plants need. Only a fraction of what is applied to the soil ends up in the crops. The rest flows to our rivers. Nitrogen and phosphorus levels, dead organisms are increasing in the Gulf of Mexico, the Rhône Delta, North Sea, Baltic Sea and Adriatic Sea. Oxygen levels fall in these coastal waters. (Phillip Lymbery 2017).

How we made a desert of the land on Earth?

Allan Savory.

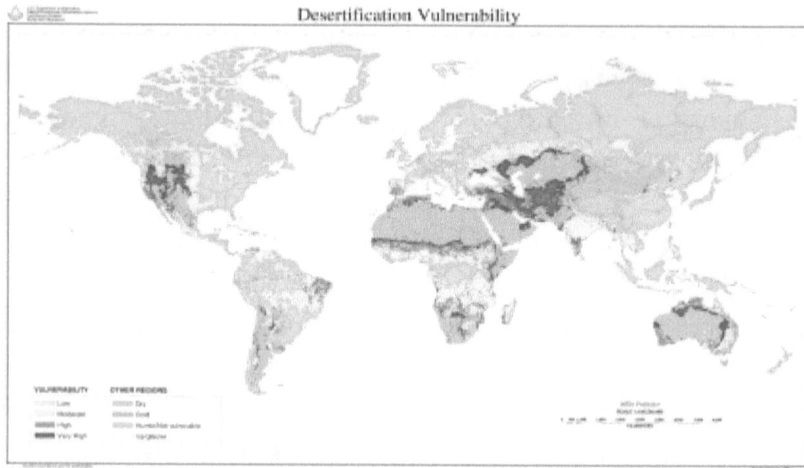

Desertification on 2/3 of the land (gray, yellow and red areas)

- When humans mastered fire, language and developed weapons like spears and axes, they were formidable predators. This was especially the case in the grasslands where their prey ran in herds. The grasslands with their deep, water and carbonaceous soils had developed for millions of years thanks to the balance between grazing animals, and the predators that fed with them.

- Modern farming methods contribute significantly to desertification and climate change due to water and air pollution from agriculture and intensive breeding of pigs, poultry and livestock. By breaking down agricultural land, we are reducing its enormous ability to retain and contain carbon.
- Chemical fertilizers to increase production have killed micro-organisms in the soil, reduced fertility of the soil and the ability to retain water and led to additional flooding. Pesticides used for the treatment of internal parasites in animals have led to the destruction of dung beetles, which are vital for soil renewal.
- Fires break the ground cover in a way that it easily carries away by rain and wind. Huge man-made deserts have arisen. **According NASA pictures from space about two thirds of the land is deserted.**
- Banks finance the farmers to rent out their pastures for solar panels and windmills and to set up even more megafarms with the aid of electrical energy.

An ever-growing meat production causes drought and hunger in large parts of the world. Fast food and an increase in meat consumption in the West are also being imitated in other parts of the world.

Rise of Man on Earth

Pan Gaia was surrounded by Pan Ocean 400 million years ago. The Earth was still a big pancake. Life on Earth has evolved in an Eastern direction under the influence of gravity, rotation of the Earth and sunlight. From Pan Ocean, the primordial soup, multicellular organisms, fish, marine iguanas and amphibians have emerged. Dinosaurs, birds, mammals and monkeys evolved on Pan Gaia. Great apes, homo erectus and homo sapiens originated in central Africa and Asia. There were no great apes on the Galapagos Islands, Easter Island, Tahiti and other central polynesian volcanic islands. North and South America were colonized from Asia not much earlier than 15,000 years ago.

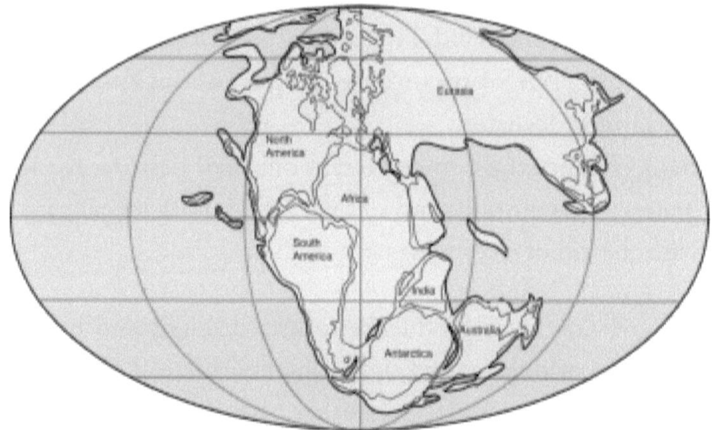

In prehistoric times there were no great apes in North and South America and therefore no homo erectus and homo sapiens.

There are howler monkeys with tails in Panama and Capuchin monkeys in the Amazon region. The original inhabitants of North and South America are from Asia. The ancestors of the modern Indians crossed during the last Ice Age, about 15 thousand years ago, from Siberia via the temporarily dry Bering Strait to present-day Alaska and from there spread mainly along the west coast across North and South America.

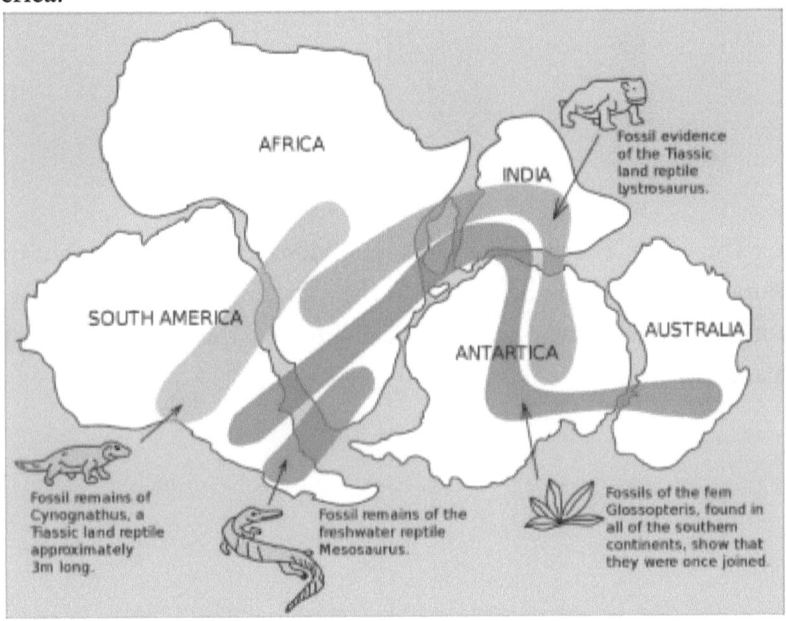

Pan Gaia, the large pancake, has spread eastward due to volcanic eruptions. This is how the five continents (North and South America, Africa, Europe, Asia and Australia) were created.

East meets West at the edges of the Great Pacific Ocean

Very ancient human civilizations have developed in the Far East.

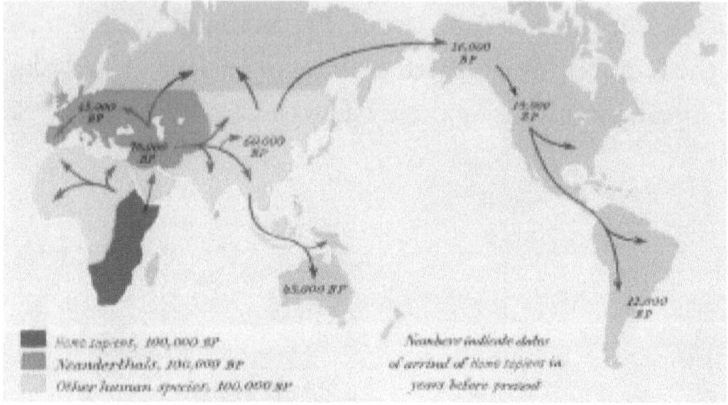

The flat Earth idea was a Mesopotamian thought that contaminated the Babylonian, Jewish, and Biblical world. That the world is spherical was mathematically demonstrated and proven later in ancient Greece.

In the Christian world, the flat Earth was systematically rejected because it was incompatible with the Bible. Hell was from below, "Heaven" from above and far on the oceans were the edges, at the risk of falling off. From the 8th century onwards, most 'Western' scholars were also convinced of the spherical shape (but they were subject to ecclesiastical silence or denial. During the first period of the Inquisition, this denial went very far. Father Abraham was said to be at the beginning of human civilization. but there were much older cultures in the Far East and even in the region of Polynesia.

At the time of Magellan and Colombus in the mid-15th century, explorers knew the world should be round, but there was no concrete evidence of this yet. Everyone (except the church) was already won over by the "round and spherical" idea at that point. The explorers still left with the idea of discovering a new world. In fact, they found in America a world with cultures that predated Rome's. Very ancient human civilizations have developed in the Far East.

There is still a large pancake - the crust that forms the bottom of the Pacific Ocean - with a rim of volcanoes that split Pan Gaia apart with their eruptions.

The Ring of Fire is still active and is generating new primitive life. 10,000 islands have been formed. There are still eruptions, the Wolf volcano in the Galapagos Islands in 2015 and the Kilauea volcano in Hawaii in 2018. Ten million years ago, late in Earth's history, the Galapagos Islands were formed. The youngest islands are the westernmost Fernandina (50,000 years) and Isabella (650,000 years). On Fernandina you even walk on the solidified lava. The marine iguanas look prehistoric. New life in the youngest volcanic islands in the Pacific, Galapagos.

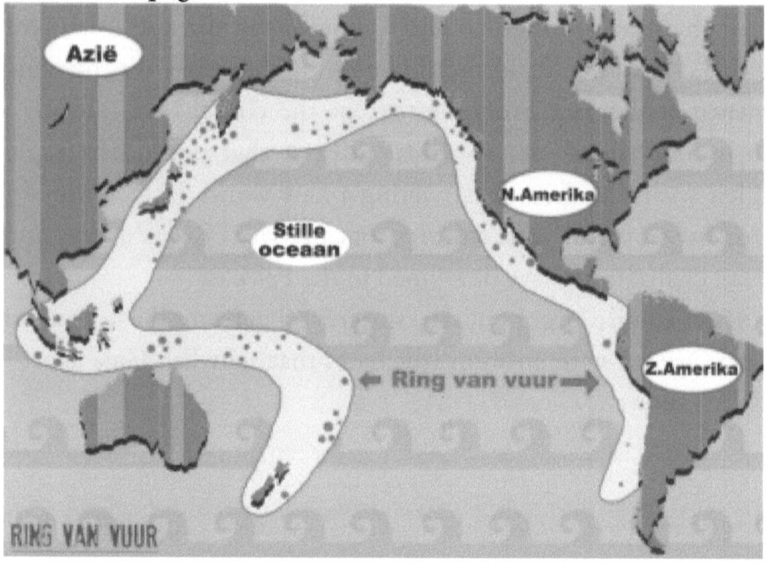

Charles Darwin (1809-1882) showed

that the finches on isolated Galapagos islands evolved under the influence of their natural environment.

Darwin: ***Environmental factors translate into physical and hereditary characteristics.***

After his comparative studies of the Galapagos Islands - The Origin of Species - Darwin wondered what his findings meant for the further evolution of life on Earth. Watson and Crick demonstrated the structure of the DNA using a double paired spiral staircase model. Achievements and qualities of the ancestors are recorded in the steps.

Humans, chimpanzees and gorillas shared a common ancestor up to 5 million years ago.

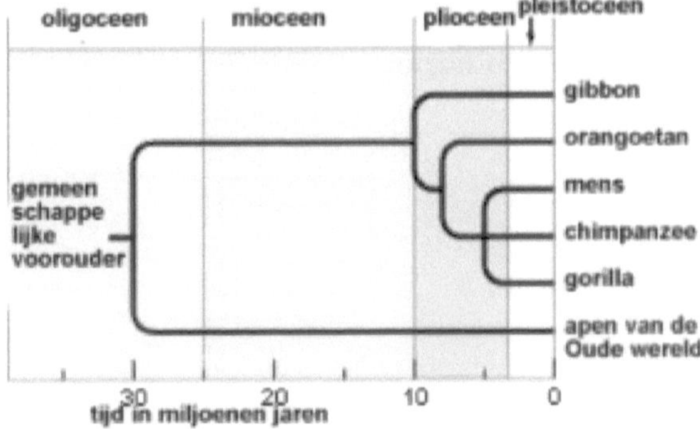

From their tree houses in Africa, the great apes have developed great manual skills. All great apes are fructivorous and feed on fruits, vegetables, nuts and beans. About a million year ago chimpanzees reached the warmer regions of Europe and Asia. From Africa via the Middle East, homo sapiens reached Western Europe 45,000 years ago. Homo sapiens has started walking upright. In that period, lions were even greater in numbers than the great apes. Neanderthals were the first to master the art of fire in Europe and have also started to consume meat and animal proteins. With wooden spears and stone axes they controlled lions, bears and other predators. Modern man has become omnivorous after this.

Great apes walk and stand on two legs. Only great apes can touch their reproductive organs with the hand. This evolution is both anatomically and functionally significant.

Chimpanzees and bonobos, in particular, became very interested in their genitalia that had come within reach.

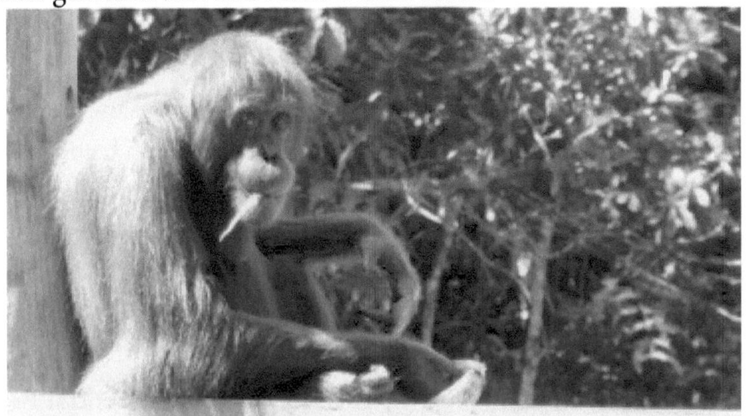

(Photo Orang Utang, Borneo)

Homo sapiens, the modern human, is at the end of the line of evolution. Only modern humans have been able to control reproduction and free themselves from the instinctual process of reproduction in the mid-twentieth century due to increased brain volume.

The rise and fall of humans on Easter Island

From Taiwan and Southeast China, three to four thousand years ago, the first brave seafarers with their double catamaran canoes with double sails, made from tree trunks and braided leaf fibers, explore the 10,000 volcanic islands in the Pacific. Thanks to their knowledge of wind, sea current and the stars, they have sailed further and further to the east.

Around 2,000 BC, these Chinese already reached New Guinea. Between 500 BC and 500 AC, the island groups of the central Pacific were colonized.

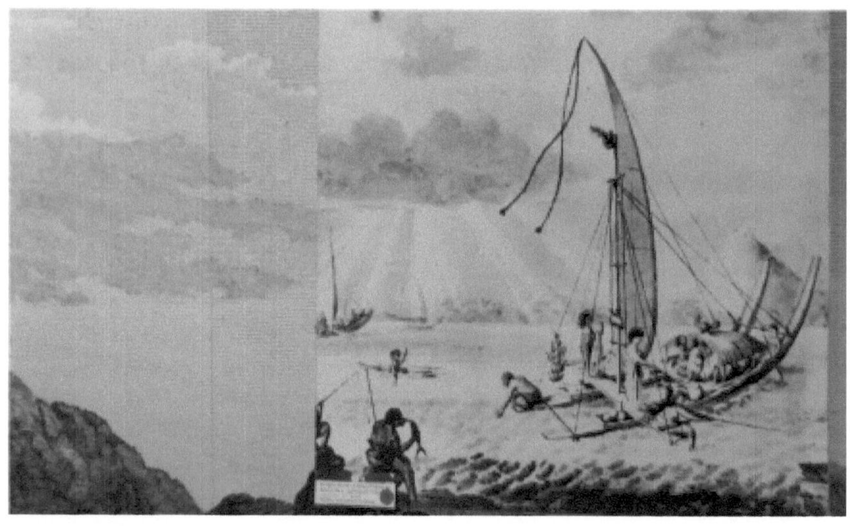

The Polynesian triangle is located between Hawaii in the north, Tahiti and its islands in the west, New Zealand in the southwest and Easter Island in the east.

- **The inhabitants of the Polynesian triangle, the Maori of New Zealand, the Rapa Nui of Easter Island and the Hawaiians speak a related language**

Residents of the Marquises Islands migrated from there to Easter Island. The Hawaiian Islands were between the years 500 and 700 conquered by these settlers. Easter Island has been as last about the year 700 discovered.

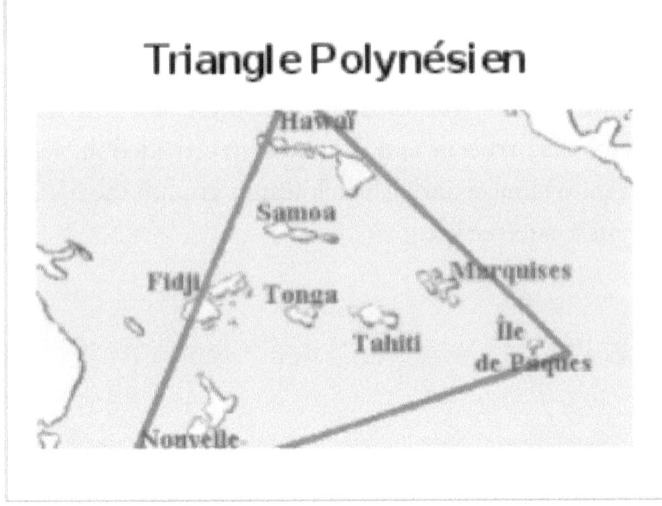

The history of humans on Easter Island began with a group of Polynesians, those from the Marquises Island around sailed east

They had brought all kinds of plants and seeds and the expedition was meant to colonize new land. New islands were found when birds were seen. Birds lay eggs on the land and their presence always means land in the neighborhood. More clouds over land are already visible from afar. These sailors also saw the pattern of the waves that an island had to be on their route. Easter Island lies 2,100 nautical miles (4,000 kilometers) after the Marquises Islands. Easter Island was uninhabited. The crater lakes in the three volcanoes contained drinking water and permanent establishment was therefore possible. They found a true paradise. The Polynesian settlers brought bananas, taro, sweet potato, sugar cane, paper mulberry, rats and chickens. The island was completely covered with palm trees. They found raw materials to make fabrics, cords and canoes. The birds in the forest, the fish from the ocean, the rats for the barbecue and the chickens provided the residents with food. The mild climate and fish-rich waters around the island gave the new residents a carefree life.

The population on the island grew rapidly, as a result of which increasingly larger parts of the forest were cut down. After all, ten groups lived on strips of land from the sea to the interior. The higher ranks lived on the coast with the holy places and the lower classes more inland. To thank the gods and to vote favorably, the inhabitants began to build the statues (or Moai). Chinese have a strong ancestor worship. The statues are representations of their ancestors, and the presence of such a statue was seen as a kind of guardian angel for a village.

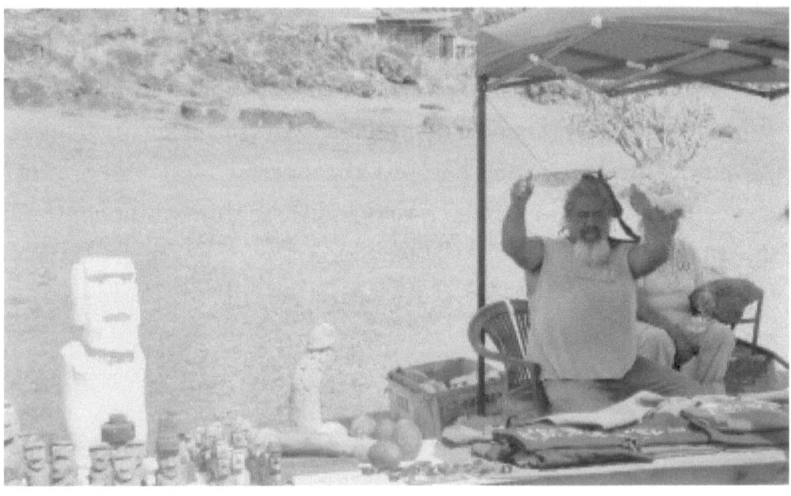

The Chinese origin of the Rapa Nui, the original inhabitants of the island is still clearly recognizable

The European discovery of the island, by the navigator Jacob Roggeveen, took place in 1722. On August 1, 1721, the then 62-year-old Jacob Roggeveen left with a fleet of the West India Company from the Reede van Texel. With three sailing ships they went in search of "The Unknown Suydlandt", a then suspected continent, which Roggeveen hoped to find with this expedition somewhere west of South America. New land, where it was thought that trading posts could be set up, was never found. On Easter Sunday, April 5, 1722, an island was first seen. They see smoke and fire and know that the island is inhabited. Since that time, this island has been called Easter Island. It turned out that the island had been inhabited in complete isolation for 1,000 years by Polynesians, who never again made the 2,000-nautical-mile journey back to the nearest land. According to Roggeveen's description, between two and three thousand people lived on the island.

It is certain that there were as many as 10,000 to 15,000 residents in the 16th and 17th centuries. The population of Easter Island had already fallen dramatically during the 100 years before the arrival of the Dutch due to the overpopulation of the extremely isolated island with its limited natural resources. There may have been a period of extreme drought with disappointing harvests and water shortages. Palm trees have been cut for farmland, for homes and canoes, and for transportation of the Moai. Rats can have a dramatic effect on a palm tree forest by eating the seeds of the plants, in this case the palm trees, preventing renewal of the forest. Rats were already present at the Polynesian colonization of the island long before Europeans discovered the island. The rats did speed up the deforestation process. Before the arrival of the Dutch, there was already a dire shortage of basic necessities. The chiefs took care of their tribesmen, but these shortages since the mid-17th century have sparked tribal conflict with even cannibalism.

The island is of volcanic origin. As big as the Dutch island of Texel.

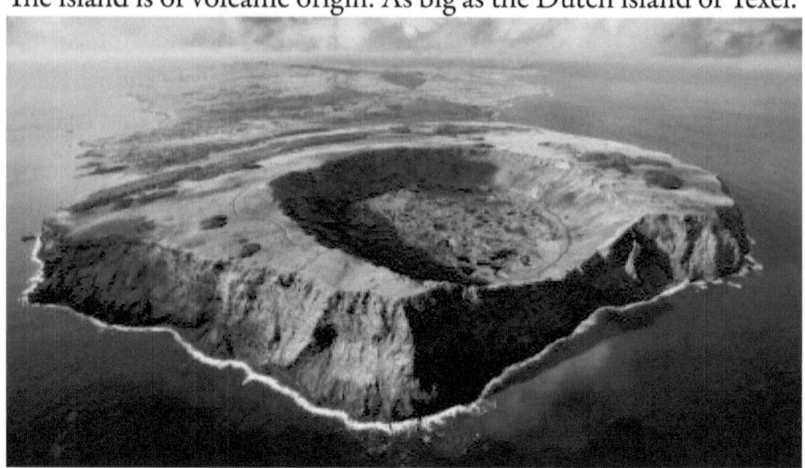

There are volcanoes on the three corners of the island: Poike, Rano Kao and Maunga Terevaka. Of particular note is the easternmost volcano that is part of the Terevaka, the Rano Raraku. Almost all the statues of Easter Island are made from the rock of this volcano. Volcanoes have made the island and images have been made of the volcanoes. The Moai statues were transported upright and carted by the population with ropes to their location. This theory ties in well with the popular legend that the Moai statues themselves walked to their place.

The Polynesians called their island "The Navel of the Wold" (Te Pito O Te Henua). Later the name "Rapa Nui", meaning big rock, became common. At the arrival of the Dutch the island was already bare and virtually treeless.

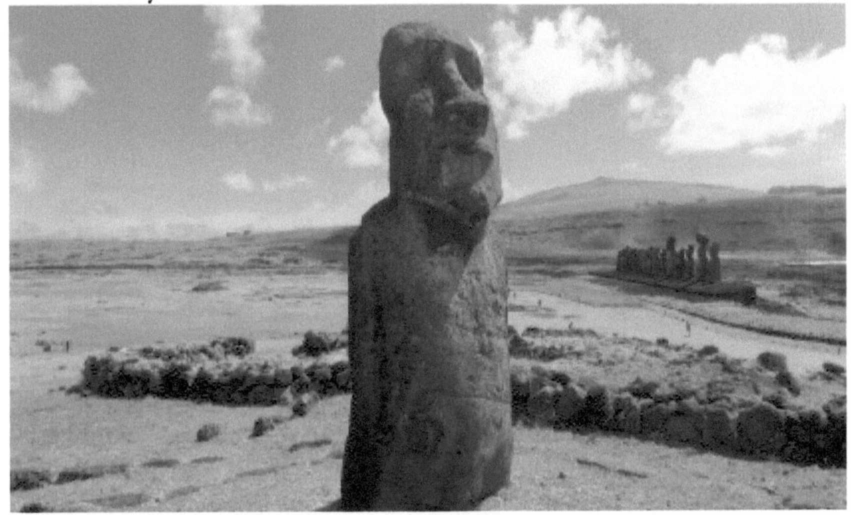

Moai

The large stone statues, Moai, for which Easter Island is world famous, were carved later than initially thought. Archaeologists now estimate that they were made between 1600 and 1730. The latter was carved around Easter 1722 that Jakob Roggeveen discovered the island. There are more than 600 large stone carvings on the island. Although the statues are often identified as "detached heads", the statues are actually full torsos.

Many Moai are buried up to their necks. Most of the statues were carved in the Rano Raraku quarry. The quarry appears to have been abruptly abandoned there, with hald-curved statues left in the rock.

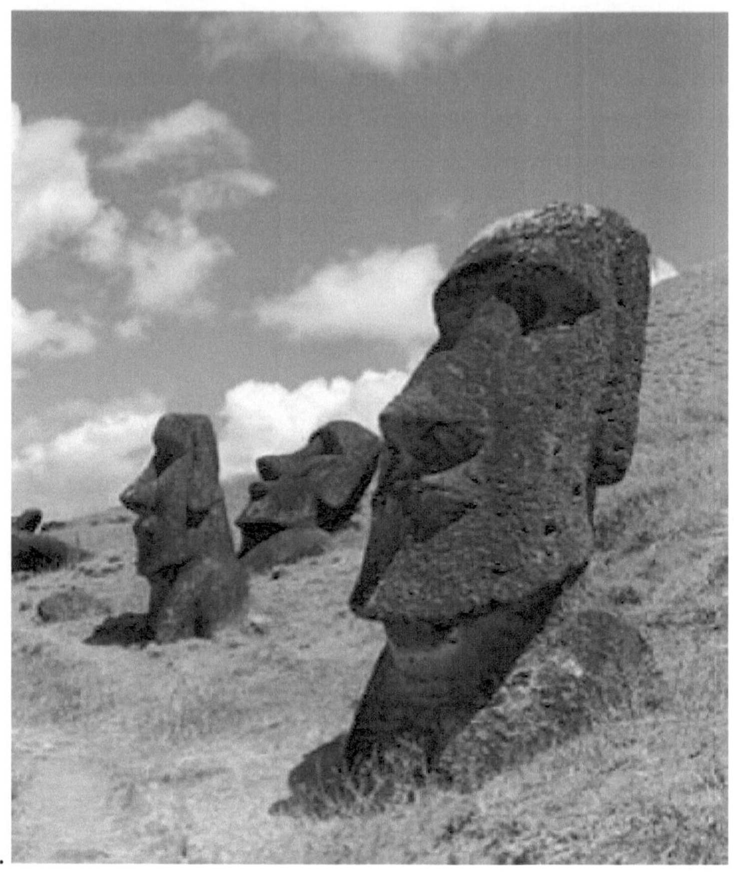

A common theory is that the statues were carved by the Polynesian inhabitants (Rapa Nui) at a time when the island was still largely covered with trees and there were sufficient resources to support a population of 10,000-15,000 Rapa Nui. Most Moai were standing statues when Jakob Roggeveen arrived. Captain James Cook saw standing statues as well as downed statues when he landed on the island twenty years later in 1744. The last European mention of an upright statue was in 1838. In 1877, the population of Easter Island was only 110 people. These 110 Rapa Nui had only 36 descendants, and they are the ancestors of all 2,296 Rapa Nui currently living on the island. In 1888 the island was annexed by Chile, so today there are about 4,000 Chileans on the island. It has been determined by decree that only the original inhabitants, the Rapa Nui, may own land on the island.

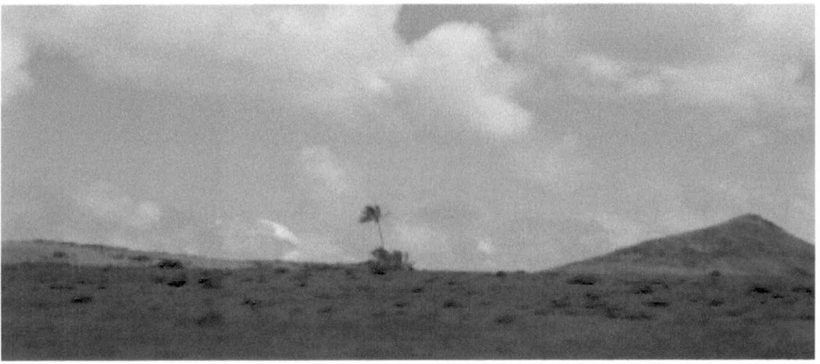

A single palm tree remained

Overpopulation

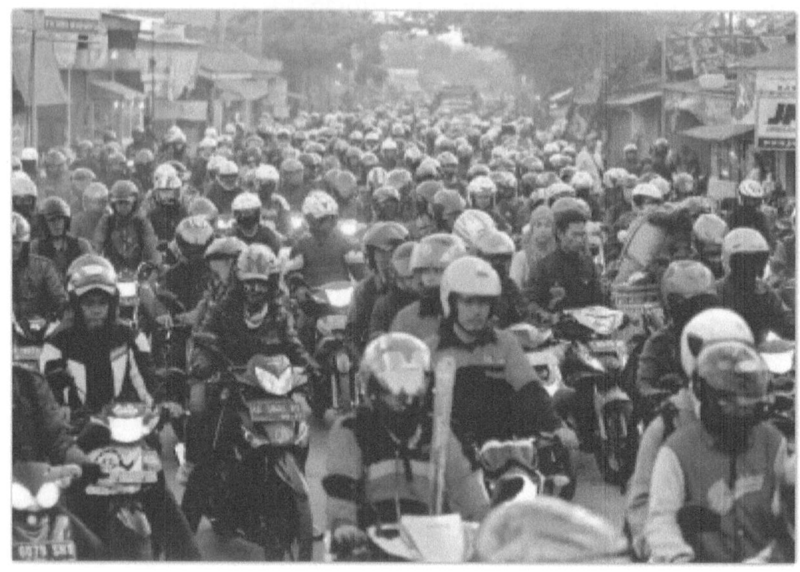

Half of the population in Indonesia is younger than 15 years

- Young people take care of elderly. Many children can take care of their retirement in the absence of a pension.

When prosperity increased in Europe, the dependence on the elderly decreased and the population increase declined. In Singapore, the two-children policy began in the 1970s. Due to the enormous influx of immigrants, the population grew, but the indigenous population growth decreased.

The one-child policy of China led to a population reduction of three hundred million people. Birth control is most common in China, with 83% of the population using one of the available contraceptives. Slightly less in Europe: 77% - and in North and South America 75%.

In Africa, the percentage is shockingly low in some countries. Contraception is expected to increase by 2030 from 17 to 27 percent in West Africa, from 23 to 34 percent in Central Africa, from 40 to 55 percent in East Africa, and from 39 to 45 percent in Melanesia, Micronesia and Polynesia (Trends in contraceptive use worldwide, 2015 United Nations).

Countries with still extreme population growth are Brazil (fifty million inhabitants in 1950, more than two hundred ten million in 2018) and Indonesia (Java in 1960 sixty million inhabitants, one hundred and sixty million in 2018). Africa, now good for one fifth of the world's population, will be the only continent whose population will continue to grow after 2050. The UN expects that by 2100 40 percent of the world will be Africans.

- **If women in Africa, who want to keep learning and work hard for more prosperity for their families, could get free contraception, the increase in the population here could also decrease.**

Part Two – Save Our Selves and Protect Planet Earth

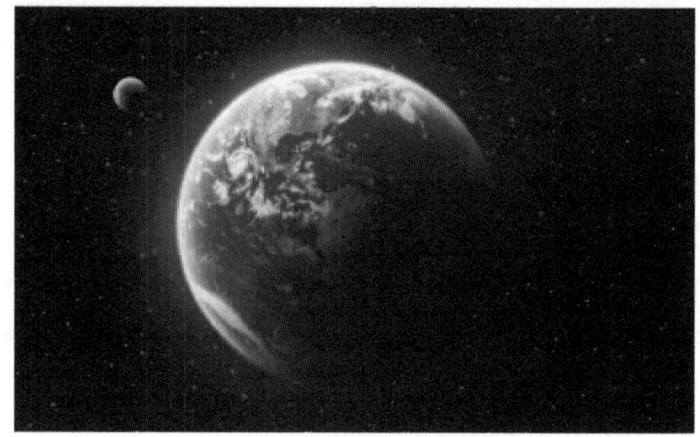

S. O. S.

Save Our Planet Earth

Fruit farmers can save the earth by changing our eating habits.

After the Spanish flu (Influenza H1N1 pandemic, originated from the poultry industry), which ruled from 1918 to 1920, due to pandemic measures the economic situation was bad, schools and resorts were closed. An economic crisis also followed in the interwar period. After World War II, the United Nations was established to define land and human rights. Later human slavery was abolished.

Will there be an economic crisis with many deaths after the second wave of Coronaviruses from 2019 to 2021 (pandemic originated from the meat industry)? The climate crisis seems inevitable and there is a great loss of plant and animal species. Will humans gain insight and abolish the slavery of wildlife and food animals?

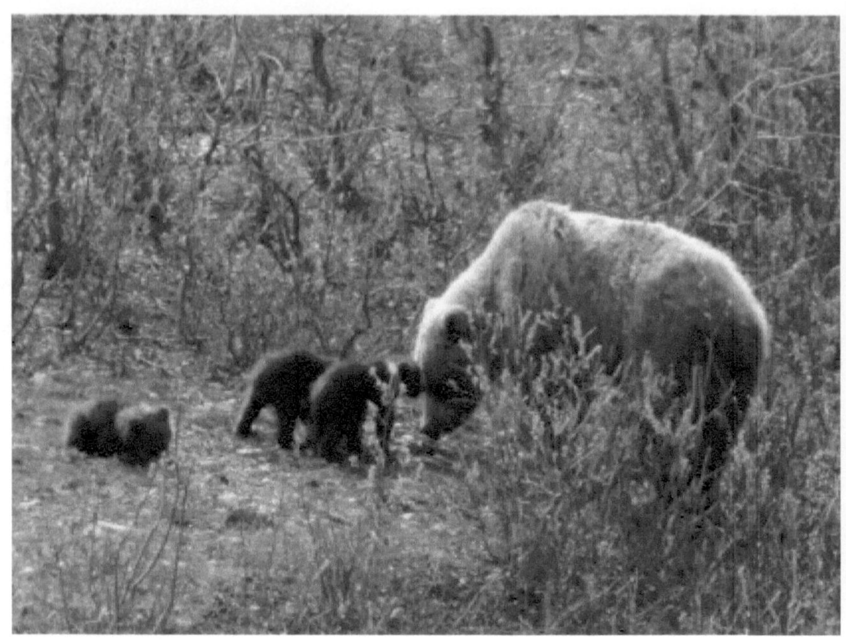

Boar with three young in Denali tundra wilderness

All mammals must have the opportunity to care for their offspring themselves. Artificial insemination of livestock and factory farming of cows, goats, pigs, sheep and rabbits is a gross violation. All mammals have a basis of life and the right to live without cruel treatment and prolonged detention.

Grasslands and grazing animals have an enormous ability to hold carbon. Agriculture can produce better vegetable and fruit as food for humans than the corn and soybeans with which we now fatten and confine the animals in factory farms to be eaten by humans.

Contraception

To put an end to the abuses in the Kempen that physician Ferdinand Peeters encountered in his daily practice, he went in search of a means by which the woman, for the sake of life, could arrange her own fertility. The contraceptive pill Enovid put on the market by the American biologist Gregory Pincus in 1957 still had too many side effects and was only admitted as a remedy for painful periods. In 1959, Dr. Peeters started a series of clinical tests with a hormone preparation offered by the German company Schering AG from his lab in the Sint-Elizabeth hospital in Turnhout. For six months, Dr. Peeters and his assistants Reimond Oeyen and Marcel Van Roy tested the preparation on fifty Kempen women for whom even more children posed a major health risk. After numerous experiments to find the right (more than half lower) dose of the two hormones (progestin and estrogen), in 1960 Peeters explained the findings to Schering in Berlin. The results were amazing. Not one of the women became pregnant and there were hardly any side effects.

After Peeters' preparation (SH 639) was found to be safe and efficient in the United States, Japan and the United Kingdom as well, Schering markets the Anovlar pill in January 1961.

Pincus tacitly acknowledged the superiority of Peeters' pill by halving the dose of Enovid in July 1961. In the end, it was Pincus who took the credit and (erroneously) went down in history all over the world as the inventor of the contraceptive pill. For fear of being robbed by the Church, however, the very Catholic Peeters did not give much publicity to his invention.

Moreover, the pioneering research of a 'rural doctor' also aroused a lot of contempt among jealous professors from the KUL where Peeters was also active.

- For centuries, sheep intestine and since 1844 Goodyear rubber has been used as a contraceptive.
- The pill, IVF and artificial insemination brought the breakthrough in the middle of the twentieth century.
- The German company Schering AG put the Anovlar pill on the market in January 1961.
- The pill proved to be a particularly powerful emancipatory agent, both in America and in Europe. The pill radically changed the balance of power between men and women - and with it the entire society.

The discovery of the pill was a great revolution. For the first time in human history, sexual intercourse and reproduction could be technically and artificially separated. The enormous commercial success was blinding, both for medicine and for theology. And everyone tried to outdo the other in giving good justification for birth control. Contraception caused a radical break with the lives of all previous generations and civilizations. Legal abortion has since been introduced, the number of divorces has increased spectacularly, euthanasia has been advocated if life is no longer experienced as meaningful. The family as the basis of church and society has crumbled into all sorts of free living together. All forms of sexuality are then openly discussed. The emergence of gays, Me Too for unwanted intimacies, sexual intimidation and rape, incest and pedophilia, gender change of transgender people, genital mutilation in other cultures. The sexual abstinence of the celibacy also had its problems such as pedophilia in priests.

Yet the balance of sudden sexual freedom is positive overall, thanks to the increased emancipation of women and the awareness of sexual problems and liberties that have been hidden for years. There are more and more women in managerial positions. We are waiting for the first woman as pope, now that women have also been admitted to church. In the metropolis of Guangzhou (the former Canton), our guide pointed us to a female Buddha in the largest temple.

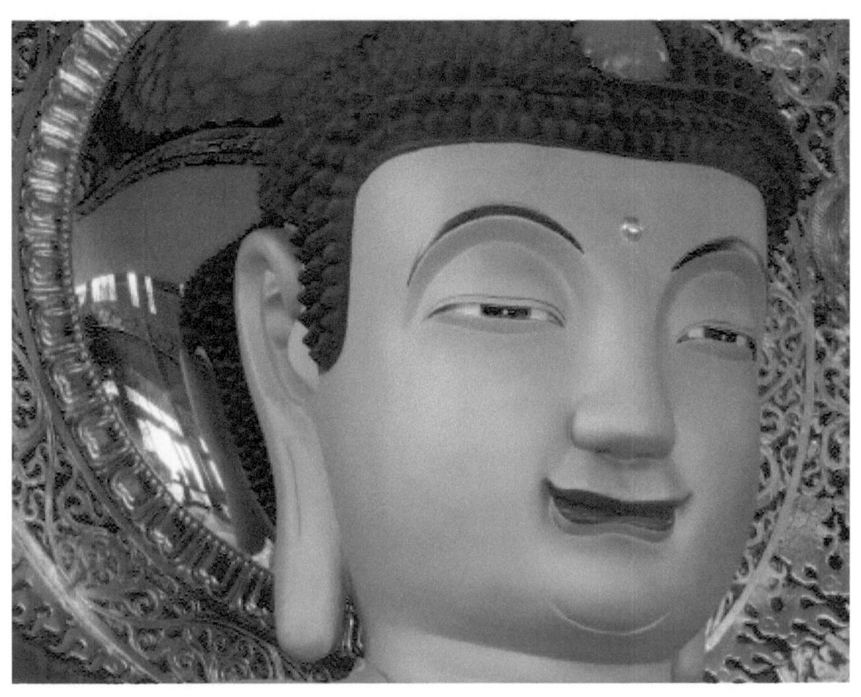

What does the sun give us?

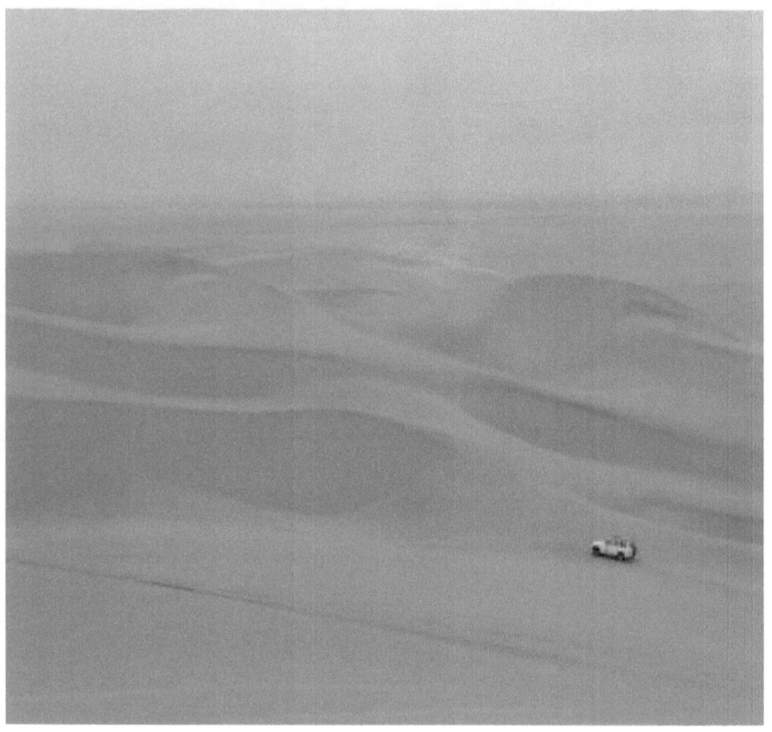

The Namib desert is one of the sunniest places in the world.

In 54 minutes, the sun drops to the earth the amount of solar energy that the whole world consumes in one year. All free renewable energy. Only it is in the wrong place at the wrong time in the wrong form. If we turn all that energy, which is now lost daily, into hydrogen, the scarcity of energy is over.

The Namib desert at Lüderitz, a port on the Atlantic Ocean on the south-west coast of Namibia, is one of the sunniest places in the world. This desert is 200 km wide and extends 2000 km from Angola in the North to the Orange River in the South along the Atlantic Ocean. In this 81,000 km2 a suitable area for energy production can be found. A combination of solar panels and hydrogen gas production with transport to the sea can offer economic benefits to Namibia.

Groningen can also earn from the transition to hydrogen gas. The Netherlands already has an extensive gas network from Groningen to the rest of the Netherlands. This natural gas network can be used for hydrogen gas transport without too much adaptation

Veendam has the first larger hydrogen plant in the Netherlands that uses solar power. It is an important step in Groningen's mission to develop into the hydrogen province of the Netherlands. Renewable energy from the electricity grid and 5,000 solar panels on the site provide green electricity to the plant, which can convert one megawatt of sustainable electricity into hydrogen. A hydrogen industry in Groningen can supply the large amounts of energy that will be lost when the oil and gas era is closed. All this energy can be stored in the form of hydrogen and transported through the gas network and in liquid form by ship.

Every day that we do nothing with the storage of solar and wind energy here and there in the Netherlands and in the deserts is a lost day. We will be saying goodbye not only to fossil fuels, but also to biofuels. The demand for palm oil has risen so much what is largely due to western policy to stimulate the use of biofuels. Fires has become increasingly fierce in recent years in the Brazilian Amazon forest and in the Indonesian tropical rainforests of Borneo and Papua New Guinea. The 'slash and burn' method (felling and burning) is used to cultivate natural land for palm plantations. Hydrogen as prime energy source could be the solution.

Canadian engineers have found a way to produce hydrogen relatively easily and cheaply from oil fields and tar sands.

By injecting oxygen into the tar sands, the temperature in the soil appears to rise. As a result, hydrogen gas is released from the oil, which can be separated from other gases by special membrane filters. Even with oil fields that are still in use, this technique can be used. A polluting fossil resource can thus be given a new lease of life and produce the energy carrier of the future. Hydrogen production is a cost-effective alternative to energy production from oil fields and tar sands. By placing hydrogen filter membranes in the production sources, only the hydrogen is extracted and undesirable by-products such as carbon dioxide diode and methane remain in the soil.

The existing infrastructure and distribution channels around the oil fields would suffice, keeping production costs low. At the moment it costs about 2 dollars to produce a kilo of H2, but with the new method that would only be 10 to 50 cents. The necessary oxygen can be produced on site. This requires no more than 5 percent of the energy produced.

Researchers from the University of Waterloo in Canada have also developed a new fuel cell that lasts at least ten times longer than current technology. These fuel cells will therefore be much cheaper.

Dutch engineers made hydrogen from sodium borohydride.

H2Fuel, a sodium-borohydride compound, is the carrier of hydrogen. The chemical name is NaBH4 (powder) and can be stored indefinitely under normal atmospheric conditions. To release the hydrogen, Ultra-Pure Water (UPW = fully pure H2O) and a little dilute hydrochloric acid are added in a certain ratio and the hydrogen molecules of both the NaBH4 and H2O are released. A total of 8H, more than 95% of the theoretically feasible amount of hydrogen is actually extracted.

(Process 1 production of hydrogen from H2Fuel)

During production, storage, transport and consumption, H2Fuel is completely free of any harmful emissions. This process, with a very high efficiency (98%), was validated by TNO Delft.

The residual product (Spent fuel, NaBO2) can later be converted back into NaBH4 in a chemical process. NaBH4 is produced in a continuous process with the spent fuel and half of the generated hydrogen gas (4H). The energy required for this can be supplied by solar and/or wind energy. As a result, the Boron and Sodium is reused very efficiently.

(Process 2 production of NaBH4)

On **sea-going vessels** osmosis allows UPW to extract fully pure water from seawater and space is available for this type of power plant.

The **Hyundai NEXO** is equipped with a 156-liter compression tank (700 bar) with hydrogen gas and has a range of 666 km. The high vehicle weight (1814 kg) comes at the expense of acceleration. With a 60-liter normal tank with sodium borohydride powder slurry, a hydrogen car can be much lighter and have a range of 700 km (2.5 times larger with the same amount of hydrogen).

A greenhouse complex in the Westland wants to be able to produce energy-neutral fruit and vegetables all year round with the help of a hydrogen power plant. Vans can be converted into hydrogen cars, and can refuel at the greenhouse complex. The spent fuel can be upgraded with solar/and or wind energy. Farmers can give their warehouses a new destination. With local production with a greater supply and diversity, the current supply of fruit and vegetables over the equator will be able to decrease.

Part three – Stay Healthy

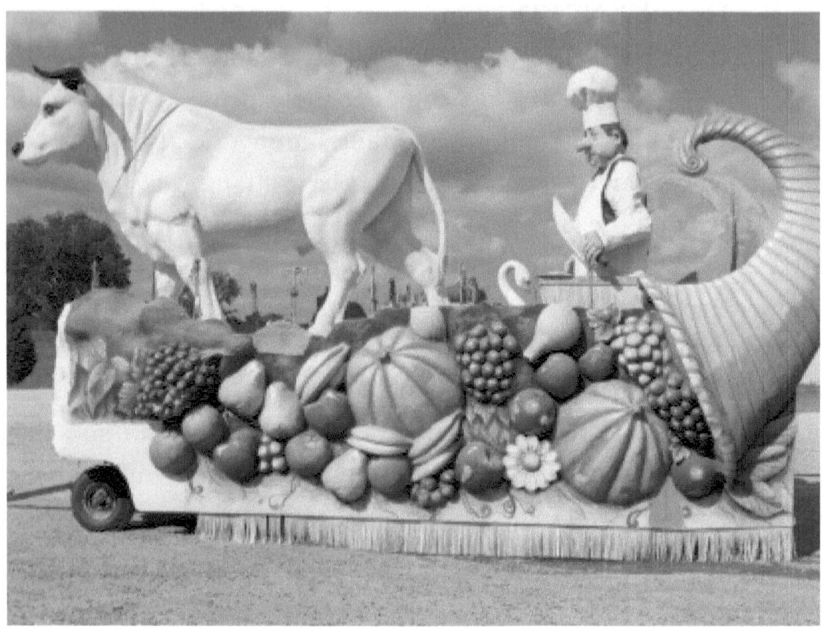

This Mardi Gras float represents the deeper meaning of Carnival - carnem levare (Latin), *let meat and eat an abundance of fruits and vegetables*

Stay Healthy for 100 years

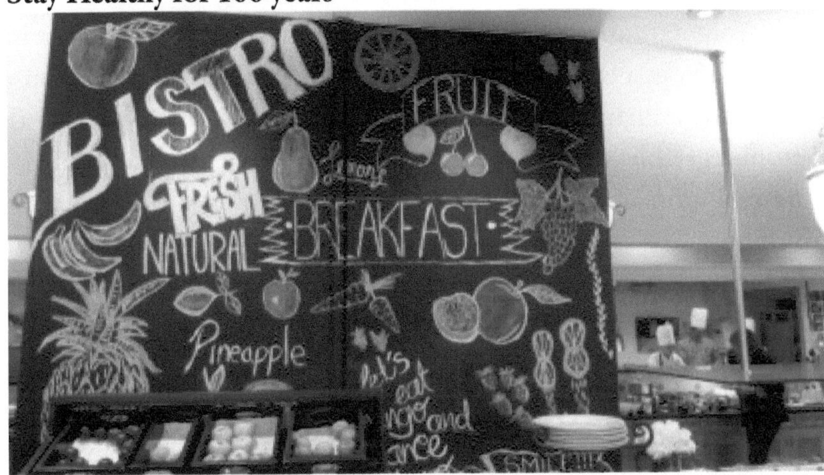

We eat everything that tastes good. If it is cheap and tasty, it also accelerates chronic disease and tumor formation. This is how our food system works. The raw materials for factory preparation are limited. Soy, corn, eggs, refined sugars, animal proteins and trans fats. These are the main ingredients that the largest food companies use to make the food that is all around us. It is not that these big companies do not care. In fact, it is difficult for them to do something else. In parts of the world with less chemical agriculture, less factory food processing, mortality from cancer is lower. Fruit and vegetable make bio-active substances that delay the growth and propagation of intruders.

Plant-based nutrition works life-extending

Voluntary diet through starvation will probably never gain much popularity as a life-prolonging strategy and is risky in connection with the development of deficiencies. Vegetable proteins - especially those from vegetables or nuts - contain less methionine than animal proteins. Several animal studies with methionine restricted diet have shown inhibition of cancer cell growth and prolonged healthy life span in experimental animals. American researchers have looked at 30 years of nutrition data among 130,000 people. They found a reduced risk of premature death in those who ate more vegetable protein and a higher risk in those who ate more animal protein. Each increase of 3% more vegetable proteins in the diet reduced the risk of death, by whatever cause, during the period under review by 10%. A link was also shown with a 12% lower risk of death from cardiovascular disease. But a 10% higher share of animal proteins in the diet led to a 2% higher risk of death and 8% higher chance of dying of a heart problem (Song M).

Unnatural nutrition is the cause of deficits and chronic diseases. Fast food, many meat products and little fruit and vegetables weaken the natural defenses. How can one switch to strictly natural food?

Oatmeal flakes

Whole grain is an important source of antioxidants and bioactive compounds such as phenols, flavonoids, and carotenoids. Flavonoids work very well as an antioxidant and prevent the conversion of calories into fat. Thus, they also have a protective effect on the blood vessels. The majority of the health-promoting compounds of whole grain are present in the germ and bran.

Vitamin C

Vitamin C is necessary for the construction of connective tissue proteins. Deficient production of these connective tissue proteins weakens the blood vessels with bleeding as a result.

Due to the frequent use of pesticides in agriculture, the content of bioactive antibodies in fruit and vegetables has been reduced, as a result of which our defense against cell infections is even more affected. Vitamin C 1000 mg protects against colds and the possible infections that accompany a cold. It was also shown that patients who took 2 grams of vitamin C per day spent a shorter time in the ICU. Patients who received vitamin C required significantly less time on ventilation.

Hemila H, Chalker E Vitamin C Can Shorten the length of stay in the ICU A Meta-Analysis. Nutrients (2019) 11(4):708

Vitamin D3 (cholecalciferol) is the precursor of the powerful steroid hormone calcitriol, which has widespread actions throughout the body. Several studies have shown that vitamin D deficiency increases the risk of developing cancer and that intake of vitamin D3 can be an economical and safe way to reduce the incidence of cancer and improve the outcome of cancer treatment. Sufficient vitamin D also increases bone density, reducing the risk of fractures.

Curcuma

Curcuma is the spice that turns curry powder yellow. In areas where this herb is eaten daily, a number of cancer diseases that are very common in Western Europe are less common.

Multiple myeloma (Kahler's disease) is a cancer of the cells of the bone marrow. This cancer is rare in India (blue area) and a lot in Western Europe (red area in the accompanying image). Plasma cells in the bone marrow ensure the production of antibodies against viruses and bacteria.

Herbs and fruits often contain the nutrients that fast food lacks. Numerous nutrients from plants, one of the best known is curcuma, protect against damage to the chromosomes of cells in the body. Malignant growth, in general, is due to DNA attack upon exposure to chemicals, radiation, or viruses that take possession of the host cell's DNA. Curcuma protects against cell DNA damage. Infected or damaged cells are now seen as abnormal and are removed from the body.

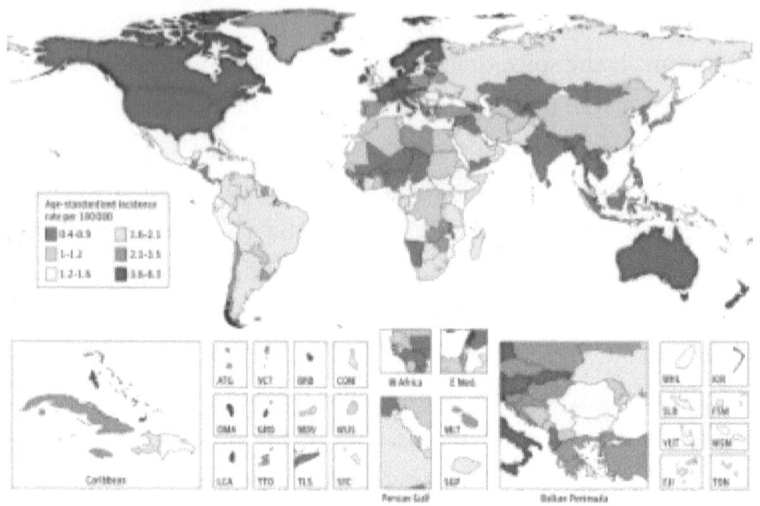

Andrew J. Cowan, Christine Allen, Aleksandra Barac et al. Global burden of multiple myeloma: A systematic analysis for the global burden of disease study. JAMA Oncol 2018 Sep 1;4(9):1221-1227

Total cancer mortality is much lower in India than in Western countries. American men get 23 times more prostate cancer than men in India. Americans 8 and 14 times more likely to develop melanoma, 10 to 11 times more colon cancer, 9 times more uterine cancer, 7-17 times more lung cancer, 7-8 times more bladder cancer, 5 times more breast cancer and 9 to 12 times more often kidney cancer than in India. This is not just 5, 10, or 20 percent, but 5, 10 or 20 times more. Indians together make up one sixth of the world's population. They have the lowest cancer rates in the world. A reduced incidence of cancer cannot be the result of increased consumption of spices alone. Several dietary factors can contribute to India's low overall cancer rates. Besides the high consumption of herbs, Indians eat little (red) meat (holy cow) and 40 percent of the Indians are vegetarians. India is one of the largest producers and consumers of fresh fruits and vegetables. Indians also eat many other spices besides turmeric. Per weight unit, turmeric contains the highest content of antioxidants (Holt PR).

Omega-3 fish oil capsules, EPA and DHA have a beneficial effect on heart and brain. Human brain cells are high in DHA. Sufficient fish in our menu is very important (Crawford MA 2012).

Benefits of Mediterranean food

The diet in Spain, Italy and Greece **is one of the healthiest eating habits in the world**. There are apparently fewer diseases here, and mortality from some chronic diseases is also less. This dietary pattern is rich in fruit, vegetables, fish, virgin olive oil and less saturated fat containing dairy products. Fats are necessary for production of hormones and the absorption of the fat-soluble vitamins A, D, E and K.

Olive oil gives food a taste and a feeling of satiety, so that you are less likely to get hungry again. This eating habit reduces the risk of cardiovascular disease, reduces the risk of diabetes, prolongs the lifespan and counts more healthy elderly people.

Avoid fast food and unhealthy trans fats

The Old McDonald's farm is very different from today's McDonald's. Fast food is in fashion. Burgers and chicken burgers are often on the menu of hard-working people. It is no longer rare for someone to go to bed with a bag of chips.

Vegetable (unsaturated) fats are liquid at room temperature and can only be processed by the food industry as a solid substance. These fats are converted into partially hardened fat by a chemical process. Products that contain partially hydrogenated fats and trans fatty acids, such as margarine, chips, cookies, coffee milk powder, tarts, crackers and pizzas are bad for blood vessels.

So, you become a hundred years

* do not fall
* do not have an accident
* do not get a cold
* do not choke, pneumonia most common cause of death for centenarians

How to stay healthy

* no colds
* do not smoke
* with clean indoor air, don’t keep birds in home
* wash hands regularly
* one glass of wine
* do not drink alcohol on a daily basis
* eat more vegetable proteins
* eat less or no red meat
* train for one hour three times a week

Burning Belly Fat

Fat burning only starts after twenty minutes of exercise. Until this time of 20 minutes, especially carbohydrate reserves (the glycogen in the liver and muscles) are burned and you will not lose weight. That is why it is better to exercise for one hour three times a week (3 x 40 minutes fat burning) than six times a week for half an hour (6 x 10 minutes fat burning). It does not matter what the training consists of. This can be brisk walking, slow jogging or a session on a treadmill or rowing machine.

Simply make your own meals

Stick to this simple advice to get rid of excess body fat and prevent diseases. Only little whole meal bread, pasta and rice to lose weight faster. Nutrition must contain many vegetables, but also sufficient vegetable proteins and fats (fish, olive oil, avocado, etc.).

- ***Start with a plant-based diet, and the need for animal proteins and fats will gradually decline***

In addition to diet, physical activity and extra antioxidant intake may counteract DNA methylation changes contributing to aging.

Fruit Breakfast

Start with two glasses of water

Oatmeal flakes with broken flax seed in soy yoghurt or soya light, almond milk or coconut milk, with fresh fruit. Like strawberries, raspberries, apples, pear, mandarin, orange, melon etc. Cut the fruit into pieces to preserve the dietary fiber.

Soup with the lunch

Make soup from vegetable broth. Think of tomato, vegetable, onion, pumpkin, mushroom, broccoli soup. A delicious soup can be made of all vegetables. Salad with nuts, mushrooms, arugula, tomato, onion, garlic, green beans, kidney beans, chickpeas etc. Olive oil dressing. Sandwich with salad of tuna, salmon, shrimp etc. or an omelet or hardboiled egg.

Omega-3 rich fish such as salmon, herring, mackerel and shellfish like mussels are much healthier than red meat.

- ***No sausages, hard-boiled eggs only, no meat (products) from the super, no insufficiently cooked BBQ meat, less dairy products, no raw milk cheese.***

Hot meal

Make especially use of herbs and spices. Replace the meat you were used to for example with chickpeas, brown or white beans. Make a delicious chili sin carne or curry dish with cauliflower, broccoli and chickpeas.

No dessert

Avoid in case of excess weight sugars and quickly digestible carbohydrates. By sweetening, the liver chooses the path of least resistance (glycolysis) and provides the requested energy, glucose, and stores excess to body fat.

Drink black coffee with a little almond milk, green tea or ginger tea after the meal. Ginger tea can be made by cutting slices from ginger root and letting it boil in boiling water. ***Alcohol and wine in moderation. The degradation product acetaldehyde is harmful to our DNA. Too many wine acids damage the esophagus and stomach.***

The farm shop and local markets

Finally, it goes without saying that for our own health we better stop the overproduction of animals for slaughter, pigs, chickens, eggs and their exports. A number of pig and chicken slaughterhouses can be closed if production is only allowed for domestic use. Farm shop and local markets are safer than oversized supermarkets. As farmers in France did, big chains like McDonald, Burger King and Kentucky Fried Chicken are better kept out now.

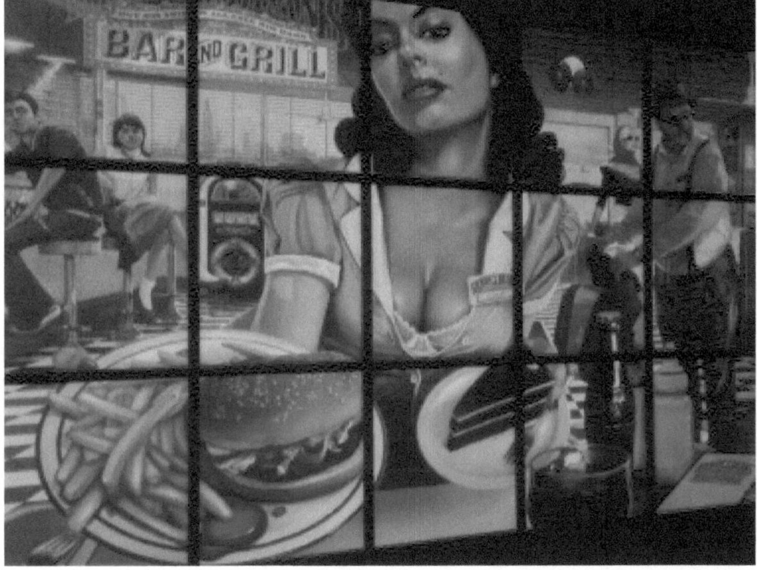

All the better restaurants nowadays also have a vegetarian menu. The farm shops could use a helping hand.

Vertical farming, multilayer cultivation

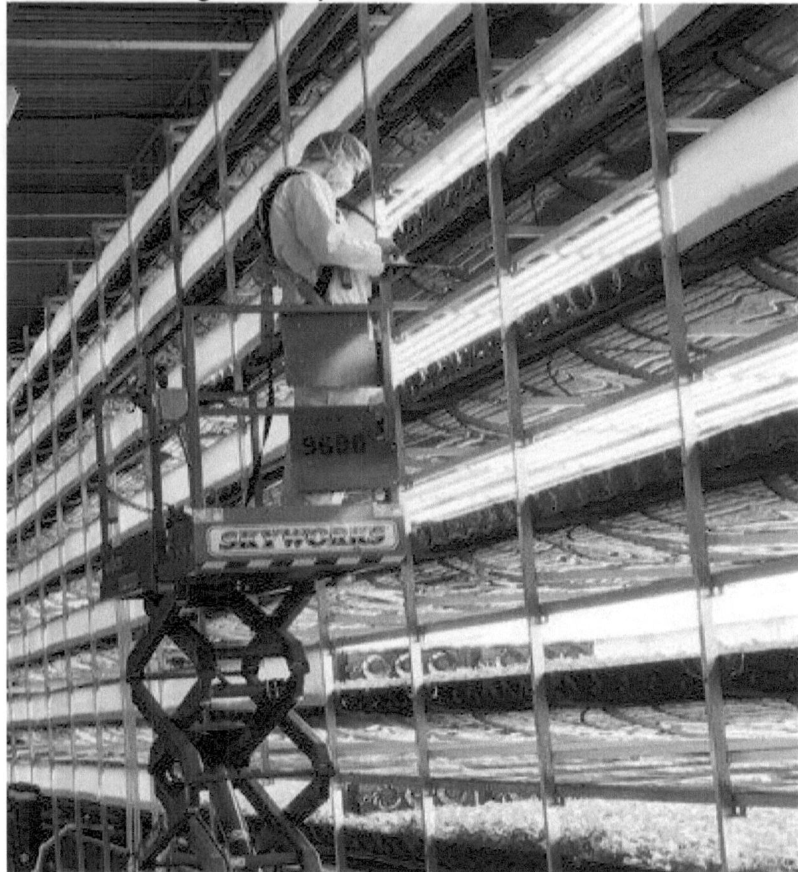

The usual agriculture and horticulture run on artificial fertilizers, pesticides and new plant varieties. Pesticides are no longer needed in a closed system.

Growing in two weeks which takes 30 days in the open ground with 95 percent less water consumption and fewer fertilizers.

Sunlight cannot be controlled. With the cooler LED lamps, which can contain all kinds of colors, engineers can develop a light recipe. They can choose the right combination of wavelengths and light intensities, place the LED lamps near the plants, and opt for wider or narrower light beams. By altering the color of lights change the smell, taste and even the vitamin content of tomatoes.

The reason for the higher yield, compared to greenhouses and outdoor cultivation, is that under LED lighting the entire plant, the whole year and long days can get enough light. In the uncontrolled sunlight, moreover, part is lost because one sheet gets too much and the other gets too little. Light is also lost due to reflection and the falling of photons on the ground.

Strawberries are sweeter and tastier when the leaves and fruit are extra lighted. In climate-controlled rooms grow in four layers among others grow lettuce, spinach, bok choy, dill or cabbage, strawberries, coriander and watercress.

In an average Dutch greenhouse, the lettuce yield is 60 kilos per square meter of floor per year. 100 kilograms per square meter shelf will be taken in the vertical shelves.

Dozens of vertical farms, also known as 'vegetable factories' or 'indoor farms', supply spinach, bok choy, dill or cabbage every day. In Miyagi, Japan, a Japanese plant physiologist ordered 17,500 LED lamps that had to be installed in a former Sony factory. This factory supplies 10,000 unsprayed lettuce heads per day. In Singapore, Panasonic opened a fully automated indoor farm for 81 tons of vegetables every year. Aero Farms in Newark, USA, opened the largest so far, a nine-meter-high warehouse that will supply 250 different unsprayed vegetables and herbs. Greenhouses are an area where machines are still surprisingly absent: picking crops such as tomatoes, peppers and strawberries has not yet been spent on robot hands on a large scale. Throughout the year, armies of pickers move into the greenhouses, which usually have relatively low wages and long and arduous working days. The picking robot is already used in Japan. In the absence of cheap labor, farmers there are in some cases satisfied with robots that harvest far less than human pickers. Even if the robot only harvests sixty or seventy percent of all strawberries, the grower earns more than if he hires relatively expensive pickers.

Agriculture on saline soils

- On Texel they succeeded in growing potatoes and vegetables on saline ground.
- Worldwide, 1.5 billion hectares of agricultural land are threatened by salinization. In areas where salinization poses the greatest threat, this offers a chance to feed families independently.
- Can the salty potato save people from the famine? Since 2010, Zilt Proefbedrijf Texel has been researching which crops grow on salty soil. Many species do well.
- The fermentation of seaweed releases 2/3 methane gas and 1/3 hydrogen gas which must only be collected and used better than the alternatives for natural gas that are currently available.

Cultured meat

The stem cells of one gram of muscle tissue can be used to make about 10,000 kilos of meat. Mosa Meat (University of Maastricht) and the Dutch food giant Nutreco are food companies that want to enter the market with lab-grown meat in 2022. They make beef from the muscle cells of a cow. The cells multiply into trillions of cells from a tiny sample. This growth takes place in a bioreactor, which is similar to the bioreactors in which beer and yoghurt are fermented. The cells are "brewed" in a liquid growth medium that includes a mixture of fats, aminos acids, carbohydrates, vitamins, and minerals. The combination of ingredients in the liquid culture prompts cells to differentiate into muscle, fat, and connective tissue.

From one sample of a cow, they can produce 800 million strands of muscle tissue (enough to make 80,000 quarters of pounds). The difference is, while it takes a cow around three years to develop enough meat to be slaughtered, we can do the whole thing in just a couple of weeks.

Global meat consumption hovers around 350 million tons per year. According to Mosa Meat, 10 tons of meat could potentially be produced from a single tissue sample. That means 35 million tissue samples would be required to satisfy the current demand for animal-based foods.

References of lung cancer studies

Anttila TI, Koskela P, Leinonen M et al. (2003) Chlamydia pneumoniae Infection and the Risk of Female Early-Onset Lung Cancer. Int J Cancer:107,681-682

Bruu AL, Haukenes G, Aasen S, Grayston JT, Wang SP, Klausen OG, Myrmel H, Hasseltvedt V (1991) Chlamydia pneumoniae infections in Norway 1981-87 earlier diagnosed as ornithosis. Scand J Infect Dis 23(3):299-304

Chaturvedi AK et al. (2010) Chlamydia pneumoniae infection and risk for lung cancer. Cancer Epidemiol Biomarkers Prev 1498-1505

Chu DJ, Guo SG, Pan CF, Wang J, Du Y, Lu XF, Yu ZY (2012) An experimental model for induction of lung cancer in rats by Chlamydia pneumoniae. Asian Pac J Cancer Prev. 2012;13(6):2819-22

Chu DJ, Yao DE, Zhuang YF, Hong Y, Zhu XC, Fang ZR, Yu J and Yu ZY (2014) Azithromycin enhances the favorable results of paclitaxel and cisplatin in patients with advanced non-small cell lung cancer. Genet. Mol. Res. 13(2):2976-2805

Coggins CR (2001) A review of chronic inhalation studies with mainstream cigarette smoke, in hamsters, dogs, and nonhuman primates. Toxicol Pathol. 2001 Sep- Oct;29(5):550-7

Felini M, Preacely N, Shah N, Christopher A, Sarda V, Elfaramawi M, Sall M, Bangara S, Gandhi S, **Johnson ES** (2012) A case-cohort study of lung cancer in poultry and control workers: occupational findings. Occup Environ Med. 2012 Mar;69(3):191-7

Ferreri AJ, Ponzoni M, Guidoboni M et al. (2006) Bacteria-eradicating therapy with doxycycline in ocular adnexal MALT lymphoma: a multicenter prospective trial. J Natl Cancer Inst 98:1375– 1382.

Ferreri AJ, Dolcetti R, **Magnino** S ey al. (2007) A woman and her canary: a tale of chlamydiae and lymphomas. J Natl Cancer Inst. 2007 Sep 19;99(18):1418-9

Ferreri AJ, Govi S., Pasini E. et al. (2012) Chlamydophila psittaci eradication with doxycycline as first-line targeted therapy for ocular adnexae lymphoma: final results of an international phase II trial. J Clin Oncol Aug 20;30(24):2988-94

Gardiner AJ, Forey AB, Lee PN (1992) Avian exposure and bronchiogenic carcinoma. Br Med J 305 :989-992

Ger LP, Liou SH, Shen CV, Kao SJ, Chen KT (1992) Risk factors of lung cancer.J. Formos Med Assoc Sep; 91 Suppl 3:222-231

Holst PAJ 1997 Risk of lung cancer needs to be studied in younger patients who keep and breed pet birds. Br Med J (1997) 314, 1353

Jackson LA, Wang SF, Nazar-Stewart V, Grayston IT, Vaughan IL (2000) Association of Chlamydia pneumoniae immunoglobin A seropositivity and risk of lung cancer. Cancer Epidemiol Biomarkers Prev 9(11): 1263-1266

Johnson ES, Ndetan H, Lo KM (2010) Cancer mortality in poultry slaughtering / processing plant workers belonging a union pension fund. Environ Res 110(6):588-94

Johnson ES (2012), Choi Km. Lung cancer risk in workers in the meat and poultry industries - a review. Zoonoses Public Health 59(5):303-13

Jöckel KH, Pohlabeln H, Bromen K, Ahrens W, Jahn I (2002) Pet Birds and risk of lung cancer in North-Western Germany. Lung Cancer Jul;37(1)29-34

Kocazeybek B (2003) Chronic Chlamydophila pneumoniae infection in lung cancer, a risk factor: a case-control study. J Med Microbiol 52(8):721-6

Kohlmeier L, Arminger A, Bartolomeycik S, Bellach B, Rehm J, Thamm M (1992) Pet birds as an independent risk for lung cancer: Case-control study. Br Med J

Koyi H, Branden E, Gnarpe J, Gnarpe H, Arnholm B, Hillerdal G (1999) Chlamydia pneumoniae may be associated with lung cancer. Preliminary report on a seroepidemiological study. APMIS 107(9):828

Laurilla AL, Antilla T, Laara E, Bloigu A, Virtamo J, Albanes D, Leinonen M, Saikku P (1997) Serological evidence of an association between Chlamydia pneumoniae infection and lung cancer. Int J Cancer 20;74(1)1-34

Littman AJ Jackson LA, Vaughan TL (2005) Chlamydia pneumoniae and lung cancer: epidemiologic evidence. Cancer Epidemiol Biomarkers Prev. 14(4):773-8

Mather JP, Roberts PE, Pan Z et al. (2013) Isolation of cancer stem like cells from human adenosquamous carcinoma of the lung supports a monoclonal origin from a multipotential tissue stem cell. PLoS One 4;8(12)

Zhan P, Suo LJ, Qian Q, Shen XK, Qiu LX, Yu LK, Song Y (2011). Chlamydia pneumoniae infection and lung cancer risk: a meta-analysis. Eur J Cancer Mar;47(5):742-7

Publications and books

Holst PAJ (1984) Bronchial carcinoma in bird keepers: an investigation in a general medical practice on a possible common relation. Ned Tijdschr Geneeskd 128:899-902

Holst PAJ, Kromhout D, Brand R (1988) Pet birds as an independent risk for lung cancer. Br Med J 297:1319-1321

Holst, PAJ (1991), Birdkeeping as a Source of Lung Cancer and Other Human Diseases. A Need for Higher Hygienic Standards.

Springer-Verlag ISBN 3-540-53555-1, Berlin/Heidelberg

Springer-Verlag ISBN 3-387-53555-1, New York

Kohlmeier L, Arminger A, Bartolomeycik S et al.(1992)

Pet birds as an independent risk for lung cancer: Case-control study. Br Med J 305:986-989

Chu DJ, Guo SG, Pan CF, Wang J, Du Y, Lu XF, Yu ZY (2012) An experimental model for induction of lung cancer in rats by Chlamydia pneumoniae. Asian Pac J Cancer Prev. 2012;13(6):2819-22.

Chu DJ, Yao DE, Zhuang YF, Hong Y, Zhu XC, Fang ZR, Yu J and Yu ZY (2014) Azithromycin enhances the favorable results of paclitaxel and cisplatin in patients with advanced non-small cell lung cancer. Genet. Mol. Res. 13(2):2976-2805

Holst, PAJ (2014) The Last Chimpanzee, somewhere in the 21st century, the last chimpanzee will die, 2014 E-book APPLE

Paperback ISBN 978-94-02124-8-4

Holst, PAJ (2015) Plant-Based food is your Best Medicine

E-book APPLE 106 pages ISBN 9789082210569

Holst, PAJ (2016) Common Cancers are Zoonoses

E-book APPLE 197 pages ISBN 978-90-824963-3-8

Holst, PAJ (2016) Increase in Cancer is a Recent Event

E-book Apple ISBN 978-90-824963-0-7

Holst, PAJ (2016) PREVENTION IS BETTER THAN CURE

E-book 978-90-824963-2-1

Hamers, RWG (2017) De tijd van de Apocalyps

Paperback 270 pages ISBN 978-9463426664

Holst, PAJ (2019) Stop the Meatballs

Paperback 131 pages ISBN 978-1797658926

Holst, PAJ (2019) Our Inheritance from the Great Apes

Paperback. 146 pages ISBN 978-1081342159

Holst, PAJ (2019) Canimalism, E-book Kindle 119 pages

Paperback 120 pages Amazon.com ISBN 978-1694357762

Hardcover 120 pages Bravenewbooks.nl ISBN 978-9402198577

Consulted books

There is much scientific evidence published and also written in several books about health benefits of plant food for several diseases in later life. Change towards strictly plant-based foods is not easy. The image of the classic vegetarian complicates this transition. But read more about the health benefits to be achieved.

The China Study

Detailed study about connection between nutrition and heart disease, diabetes, and cancer. The report also examines source of nutritional confusion produced by powerful lobbies, government entities and opportunistic scientists. The China Study observed whether there were patterns of associations for different dietary, lifestyle and disease within the survey of 65 counties, 130 villages and their families. Within this study in China and Taiwan, was also investigated the virus hepatitis B (HBV), which causes primary liver cancer, a major cause of death in Africa and Asia. They collected data on the prevalence of people having antibodies and antigens, multiple disease mortality rates, and many nutritional risk factors. HBV antibody prevalence was highly correlated with vegetable consumption, dietary fiber, and plant protein. In short, more plant food consumption was associated with more antibodies and improved immune response.

Campbell TC, Campbell TM (2006) **The China Study**. electronic Book Apple

How Not to Die

The vast majority of premature deaths can be prevented through simple changes in diet and lifestyle. In How Not to Die, Dr. Michael Greger, the internationally renowned nutrition expert, physician, and founder of NutritionFacts.org, examines the fifteen top causes of premature death in America-heart disease, various cancers, diabetes, Parkinson's, high blood pressure, and more-and explains how nutritional and lifestyle interventions can trump prescription pills and pharmaceutical and surgical approaches, freeing us to live healthier lives.

Gene Stone & Michael Greger MD

Proteinaholic, how Our Obsession with Meat is Killing Us and What We Can Do About it

Whether you are seeing a doctor, nutritionist, or a trainer, all of them advise to eat more protein. Foods, drinks, and supplements are loaded with extra protein. Many people use protein for weight control, to gain or lose pounds, while others believe it gives them more energy and is essential for a longer, healthier life. Now, Dr. Garth Davis, an expert in weight loss asks, is all this protein making us healthier? The answer, he emphatically argues, is NO.

Too much protein is actually making us sick, fat, and tired, according to Dr. Davis. The healthiest countries in the world eat far less protein than we do and yet we have an entire nation on a protein binge getting sicker by the day.

Garth Davis MD & Howard Jacobson

Guns, Germs, and Steel: The Fates of Human Societies

Guns, Germs, and Steel seek to answer the biggest question of post-Ice-Age human history: why Eurasian peoples, rather than peoples of other continents, became the ones to develop the ingredients of power (guns, germs, and steel) and to expand around the world. Africans enjoyed a huge head start, because Africa is the continent with by far the longest history of human occupation. North America is a big fertile continent, with the result that it supports the richest and most productive nation today. Australia provides by far the earliest evidence for human ability to cross wide water gaps, and some of the earliest widespread evidence for behaviorally modern humans. Why, nevertheless, were Eurasians the ones to expand? The reasons were continental differences in the available wild plant and animal species suitable for domestication, resulting in earlier more productive suite of domesticates in Eurasia.

The Eurasia's east/west axis facilitated the spread of those domesticates throughout Eurasia. Europeans were able to spread at the expense of other peoples by infecting them (usually unintentionally) with epidemic infectious diseases such as smallpox and measles, to which Europeans had evolved some genetic resistance and had acquired much immune (antibody-based) resistance through historical and lifetime exposure respectively, while unexposed non-European peoples had no such exposure, hence no such resistance. The exchange of major epidemic infectious diseases was one-sided, because most of those diseases in the temperate zones came to us humans from diseases of our domestic animals (such as cattle, pigs, and chickens) with which our ancestors lived in close contact after those animal species had been domesticated. But of the world's 14 species of valuable domestic mammals, 13 were Eurasian, only one American, and not a single Australian. Hence Eurasians ended up as disease bearers, and with much resistance themselves to their own diseases.

Jared Diamond 1997.

Dead Zone, where the wild things were

A tour of some of the world's most iconic and endangered species, and what we can do to save them. Climate change and habitat destruction are not the only culprits behind so many animals facing extinction. The impact of consumer demand for cheap meat is equally devastating. We are falsely led to believe that squeezing animals into factory farms and cultivating crops in vast, chemical-soaked prairies is a necessary evil, an efficient means of providing for an ever-expanding global population while leaving land free for wildlife. Our planet's resources are reaching breaking point.

Large amounts of nitrogen from fertilizer and manure are distributed annually over agricultural land. No doubt that it increases crop yield, but plants do not absorb it completely, so that more fertilizer and animal waste is added than the plants need. Only a fraction of what is applied to the soil ends up in the crops. The rest flows to our rivers. Nitrogen and phosphorus levels, dead organisms are increasing in the Gulf of Mexico, the Rhône Delta, the North Sea, the Baltic Sea and the Adriatic Sea. Oxygen levels fall in these coastal waters.

Dead Zone takes us on an eye-opening investigative journey across the globe, focussing on a dozen iconic species and looking in each case at the role that industrial farming is playing in their plight. Phillip Lymbery. 2017

David Attenborrough - A Life on Our Planet

Hundreds of studies around the world have confirmed that something is going on. The consequences will be more far-reaching than the pollution of the soil and water in a few countries. Ultimately, this could lead to the disruption and collapse of everything we rely on.

This is the tragedy of our time: the accelerating decline in the biodiversity of our planet. We need overwhelming biodiversity if life on our planet is really to flourish. Only when billions of different individual organisms make the best use of all the resources and opportunities they encounter, and when millions of species live interlinked lives that are interlinked in such a way that they sustain each other, can the planet function smoothly.

The greater the biodiversity of our planet, the safer all life on earth, including ourselves, will be. However, biodiversity is plunging under the influence of our current way of life.

We lead our pleasant lives in the shadow of a disaster that we ourselves are causing. This catastrophe is caused by the very things that enable us to create an atmosphere of well-being. And it is logical that we will continue to do so until we have a decisive reason to stop doing so, and an appealing alternative. The natural world is in decline. The evidence is compelling that it will lead to our destruction. There is another alternative to turn the tide if we act now. Part of the solution may lie in the Netherlands, one of the few countries explicitly mentioned in the film. Attenborough explains that it is a densely populated country but is still the world's second largest exporter of food. Attenborough shows the efficient way vegetables are grown in our country, in greenhouses and under artificial sunlight. He also points out how the Netherlands deals with seawater. One of the problems we will face with city flooding as a result of climate change. Netherlands can also teach the rest of the world a lot about that.

Acknowledgement

For the bachelor examination I did my pathology exam with Professor Dr. A. de Minjer. My thesis on small cell lung cancer was discussed and the Minjer took me to the pottery museum where they stopped for some time in front of a preparation with lung carcinoma of a smoker. De Minjer pointed that lung cancer and breast cancer for the coming years would be the biggest challenges of medicine. More than fifty years later, that is still the case.

Because of the many consultation hours and home visits, ten lung cancer patients came to my attention in the general practice. Of these, there were six bird keepers in the years before diagnosis. After consulting with professor F. de Waard of the RIVM, department of epidemiology, I have set up a ten-year practice survey and follow-up studies. The statistical link was demonstrated, later confirmed in studies in Berlin and Glasgow.

I would like to thank professor Zwart (Department of Veterinary Pathology, Division for Diseases of Special Animals. State University Utrecht) for his comments after the presentation of my research findings. "Original ideas and observations are rare. They are especially valuable if checked in practice, critically evaluated and supported by material independently collected by others.

Holst noticed a potential connection between the keeping of birds and the occurrence of lung cancer among members of households where they are kept. He has pursued the idea in his private practice and over 12 years kept records of every single patient. The data were critically and statistically analyzed and supplemented by data and materials collected by lung specialists". Research in cancer, especially in lung cancer in humans, has involved a large input of science and has contributed considerable to knowledge of the many factors involved. A new aspect is presented in avian products, spread in the house in the form of fine dust particles, inhaled deeply, cause irritation and contribute to local immune responses in the lungs. Much later, in 2012, laboratory experiments proved the link between lung cancer and Chlamydia pneumonia infection (Chu DJ 2012 & 2014).

Dr Michael Greger MD was very predictive with his publication on the emergence of zoonoses.

Greger, M. (2007). The human/animal interface: emergence and resurgence of zoonotic infectious diseases. Critical Reviews in Microbiology, 33(4), 243-299.

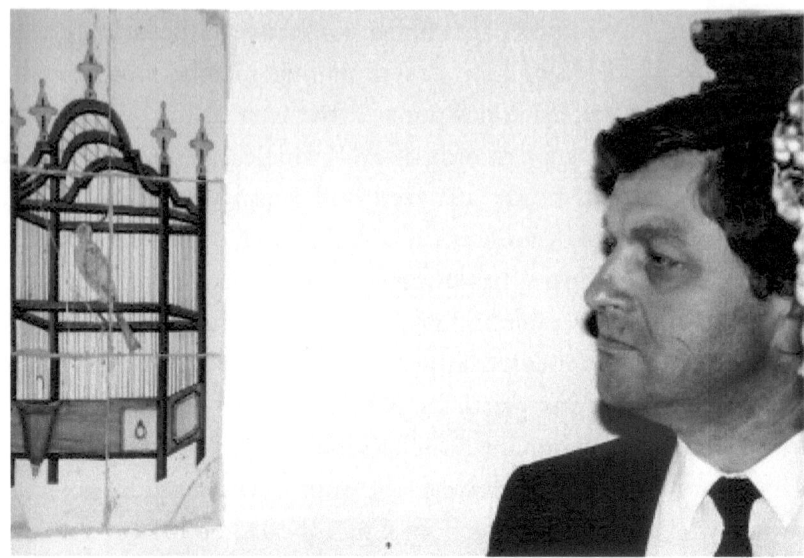

Dr. Peter Holst worked until 1984 as a general practitioner in The Hague area, the Netherlands. As a starting general practitioner in 1970 he saw a young girl with a severe case of Chlamydia pneumonia. After treatment with an antibiotic, she recovered. Because she kept a budgie in a cage in her bedroom, he assumed "the presence of a caged bird at home could be responsible for more serious disease". In his practice he also treated a 17 year of age boy with an osteosarcoma in his upper leg, where he died from. As a hobby he kept and bred about 100 tropical birds in a basement room.

Because of the many consultation hours and home visits, ten lung cancer patients came to his attention in the following years. Of these, there were six bird keepers in the years before diagnosis. After consulting a professor in epidemiology, he started a ten-year practice-survey. He did his research with the University of Utrecht. Unique by the combination of veterinary and human medicine. Diseases that from animals to humans can pass (zoonoses) are becoming more common. With support from the Dutch Prevention Fund, he did research into new cancer cases in his own practice (ten-year practice survey). The results were published in the Netherlands Journal of Medicine (Holst 1984). After this he began a case-control study of all newly diagnosed lung cancer patients in all hospitals of The Hague with the aid of their own lung specialists. The results of these studies were published in the British Medical Journal (Holst, Kromhout & Brand 1988). Bird keeping and bird breeding were proven to be a risk of lung cancer. In the study of lung cancer patients in The Hague, except the risk of keeping birds in the house, especially breeding of birds, they found also a decreased intake of vitamin C with fresh fruits and vegetables.

With the Dutch Organization for Applied Scientific Research (TNO Delft) he then carried out dust measurements in homes of bird keepers.

In 1987, this research led to his PhD at the University of Utrecht on the relationship he demonstrated between breeding and keeping birds indoors and lung cancer. He defended the hypothesis that lung cancer in bird keepers and bird breeders is the result of persistent infection of the deeper basal cells in the airways. These basal cells are still multipotent and do not die if the cell is infected with a bacterium like the Chlamydia that can only propagate in a living host cell. His promoters were prof. F. de Waard, epidemiologist of the RIVM, professor P. Zwart, head of the Veterinary Faculty University Utrecht and D. Kromhout, nutritional epidemiologist. GP studies and dust measurements with TNO were supported by the Dutch Prevention Fund.

Holst specialized from 1984 in Occupational and Environmental Health Services at the Netherlands Institute Preventive Medicine (NIPG-TNO Leiden). Since its founding in 1991, he was a member of the International Society of Indoor Air Quality (ISIAQ). He has published in various medical journals and has written books on indoor air hygiene and preventive medicine.

After his retirement in 2005 he traveled a lot. Born in Zeeland, land in the sea, he is attracted to the wide world and the tidal inlet. After more than 20 cruises, he has now crossed all oceans several times. The volcanic islands in the great Pacific Ocean are very impressive. All the first life forms originated here and spread to America, Africa, Europe, Asia and Australia. Fish, amphibians, birds, dinosaurs and mammals originated from the primordial soup of the Pacific Ocean. He noticed that there were no great apes in America and Australia. The oldest human civilizations are found in the Far East. Recent DNA research has shown that 70,000 years ago the Aborigines reached Australia from East Africa via Antarctica.

In 2012 a laboratory experiment proved the link between lung cancer and Chlamydia pneumonia infection.

His interest in the link between breeding tropical birds and cancer has expanded to the health risks of the intensive rearing of poultry, pigs and cattle for consumption. Since the fifties of the 20th century, artificial breeding in livestock has increased sharply. In the past fifty years, our diet has become increasingly unnatural. More meat products from animals, solely bred for consumption, cause more chronic diseases. An increase that keeps pace with the recent increase in cancer mortality.

www.ingramcontent.com/pod-product-compliance
Ingram Content Group UK Ltd.
Pitfield, Milton Keynes, MK11 3LW, UK
UKHW041823200726
13854UKWH00002BA/529